LOVE
IN THE TIME
OF HIV
THE GAY MAN'S GUIDE
TO SEX, DATING,
AND RELATIONSHIPS

MICHAEL MANCILLA AND LISA TROSHINSKY

THE GUILFORD PRESS
NEW YORK   LONDON

Library of Congress Cataloging-in-Publication Data

Mancilla, Michael.
   Love in the time of HIV: the gay man's guide to sex,
dating, and relationships / Michael Mancilla, Lisa
Troshinsky.
      p. cm.
   Includes bibliographical references and index.
   ISBN 1-57230-843-5 (pbk.)
   1. Gay men—Sexual behavior. 2. AIDS (Disease)—
Prevention. 3. Gay men—Health and hygiene. 4. Intimacy
(Psychology) 5. Gay men—Life skills guides.
I. Troshinsky, Lisa. II. Title.
   HQ76.M234 2003
   306.76′62—dc21
                                                    2003010341

To Jerry: Together we loved and lived our lives in the aggressive pursuit of joy.

–M. M.

To David: The positive hold you had on life emanates even in your absence and helps me to live my life completely.

–L. T.

CONTENTS

Acknowledgments   ix

Note from the Authors   xi

Preface   xiii

Introduction   1

ONE   Tell and Kiss: The Skill of Disclosure   9

TWO   Transitions: Reflection, Resilience, and Opportunity   33

THREE   Love in Contrast: Negative and Positive   59

FOUR   An Indian Summer Romance: Positives with Positives   82

FIVE   Jumper Cables and Relationships: 118
Negatives with Negatives
Mark E. Wojcik

SIX   In Sickness and in Health: 135
Your Body and Your Relationship

SEVEN   Lazarus and Survivors: Those Who Continue   164

Epilogue   201

APPENDIX A   Legal Protections for Couples with HIV   203
             Liz Seaton

APPENDIX B   Resources   215

             Notes   219

             Index   225

             About the Authors   235

ACKNOWLEDGMENTS

This book could not have been accomplished without the support of a variety of people. These include Jen Cook, who served as an early collaborator on this project, and Mark Sullivan, the former senior editor of the *New York Blade* and my friend of the last nineteen years, who provided early support and encouragement as well as critical assistance in putting together the proposal for this book. I especially value the enthusiasm and intelligent questions of my former editor, Frank Darmstadt of Insight Books, as well as Kitty Moore and Christine Benton of The Guilford Press, who mixed their own blood and sweat into the very ink of these pages.

I am grateful to Mark Wojcik and Liz Seaton, who both contributed original material as well as compassionate voices in their understanding of the virus.

Thom Collins, whose photo graces the cover, presents a beautiful face and body, as well as spirit, to those of us living with HIV.

For their support, friendship, advice, love, and help with specific information, I thank Ivan Ortiz Torres and my former colleagues at the DC Agency for HIV/AIDS and at Pride Institute; my friends Michael Lohri, MSW; David Austin; the unsinkable Delores Carter, RN; Rob Falk; F. J. Venezia; the Rev. Patty Ackerman, my spiritual touchstone during a difficult time; members of the HIV Community Coalition; my fellow board members, Cornelius Baker, and the staff of Whitman–Walker Clinic; my physician, Mary Young, MD; and, of course, my family.

I acknowledge, with warmth in my heart, my former partner

Jerry's parents, Jean and Gerald Roemer, with whom I continue to have an ongoing, caring relationship; Eric, who became a part of my existence in sailing the uncharted waters of relationships and showed it was possible to love again; and my dear collaborator, Lisa Troshinsky, who helped breathe new life into this endeavor. Her willingness to join me midstream during the interviewing process and her editorial assistance helped bring this project to fruition.

Last and most important, I thank the people who opened their hearts in sharing the stories. Although their names may have been changed by me to protect their identities, their messages of the possibilities of love come shining through.

—M. M.

Writing this book with Michael has been a wonderful experience for me and has definitely taken priority status in my life for the last year and a half.

It all started when, in between reporting gigs, I innocently answered an ad (that "had my name written all over it") looking for a "writer of one chapter for a book about HIV." That first shy meeting with Michael in a coffee shop quickly turned into my adopting the role of coauthor, and Michael and I have been a close team ever since.

And so I want to thank Michael, first and foremost, who allowed me the experience of working with him—a relationship that is precious to me on both a business and a personal level.

I also want to thank my dear friend Ajene, who has stood by me on the sidelines through all the long hours of writing and editing; and all of my English teachers and editors who told me I could write!

I would also like to remember my dear friends who died of AIDS—in particular, David Holmes, who was also my dance teacher and mentor, and who even now, almost a decade after his death, inspires me to express myself in creative ways.

—L. T.

NOTE FROM THE AUTHORS

HIV is a constantly changing disease, and references to the state of research and treatment may not be up to date by the time this book is published. Moreover, the statements and opinions in this book are not intended to replace the advice of a physician.

Likewise, descriptions of unsafe sex practices, including non-disclosure of HIV status, are observations about what is happening in certain segments of the gay community and are in no way meant as endorsements by the authors of such practices.

PREFACE

TAINTED LOVE: GM 32, attractive, who has more Aztec in his blood than AZT. This T-Cell tease is seeking an intelligent partner with a dark sense of humor, who enjoys groovy coffee shops, kite flying & ???

I placed this ad the April after I was diagnosed with HIV. Ironically, it was another personal ad that had caused me to get tested for HIV as well as started me on the journey toward this book. During the previous spring I had placed an ad beginning with "Guys seldom make passes at guys who wear glasses." (I have a weakness for intelligent-looking men.) On a summer afternoon with my nearsighted friend—the memory is ingrained because the moment has a clarity that comes from both sunshine streaming through the window and life-changing significance—the condom broke. If panic can have both an intelligent and a rational component, I believe this is how we responded to this personal crisis. We both agreed to be tested and to share the results with one another.

I went to the local Public Health Department, was given a nonidentifying number, had my blood drawn, and was given a lecture in a bored tone on safer sex practices that I could have recited myself. Within two weeks my friend received negative results. This brought me a smidgen of hope and relief as I considered my own HIV status. Because of my clinical training as a therapist, I know how I am supposed to feel, how I am supposed to react to problems in a healthy manner, but facing an emotional crisis with someone I am involved with presents a different challenge all together.

The day I drove to the clinic the leaves had already changed.

On this vivid Indian summer day I made my deal with God, only mine was reversed. Without specific expectations from creation I promised that if the test was positive, I would commit my life to working with other HIV-positive people; if the test was negative, I would continue working with troubled adolescents.

The counselor's eyes gave it away as they filled with sorrow and compassion. "I'm sorry," she said. "It came back positive."

I do not think I ever went into denial about being HIV positive. It seemed that too much time would be used by it, and time was something I could not spare. Later I found in what moments of sadness I experienced an opportunity for reflection and peace that can only come through melancholy. Two months later, true to my deal with God, I got a job working at the city's agency for HIV/AIDS. There, as a clinical social worker, I would provide direct psychotherapy and case management for the clients who, like me, were facing this virus. (See the accompanying box.)

Throughout the winter I began the process of redefining myself as a prospective romantic and sexual partner. Celibacy had no more appeal than before my diagnosis, but figuring out how to reveal my status to others was a challenge. I went out on the weekends to my regular haunts, the gay bars and parties, but disclosure in these environs was tricky. Nothing is more quick to dampen a budding erection than a sympathetic hug and an offer of friendship. I moved on to attend parties for HIV-positive men and to cruise auditoriums during medical workshops. I even struggled with my attraction to a member of a support group I was running. The rules forbade dating within that small circle, and being the therapist for the group confounded the issue.

Finally I returned to the personals and placed the ad reprinted above. Neither the local *City Paper* nor the *Washington Blade* would print my ending,

> The Centers for Disease Control and Prevention (CDC) recommend annual screening for HIV, chlamydia, syphilis, and gonorrhea for gay and bisexual men, as well as vaccination against hepatitis A and B. The CDC notes that some men in high-risk groups may need to be screened more often. For counseling and testing sites in your area, contact your local AIDS Service Organization, Public Health Department, and in the United States call 1-800-342-AIDS(2437), or via the web, *www.ahstd.org*.

"searching for someone to redefine the term 'night sweats,' " replacing it with the question marks. I can only wonder at the reasons. Are HIV-positive folks not supposed to be sexy? Not supposed to have sex? Regardless of the omission, I was pleasantly surprised by the number of responses I got. HIV-negative, -positive, and untested men were interested in me. I even met someone who just really liked Soft Cell's version of the song "Tainted Love" and had not immediately caught on that I was HIV positive. Even though the personal ad did not provide me with a partner, it helped me begin to define myself as a romantic and sexual being with HIV.

In this process I have also come to identify myself as both healer and patient. In my private practice I continue to hear about the issues and challenges of dating and relationships with HIV. The themes familiar to those of us who work with people living with HIV—of illness, acceptance, and loss—now require new responses that challenge our creativity and compassion and are more imbued with hope. In my personal life, I have continued to keep a calendar not only of my doctors' appointments but of dinner dates and anniversaries as well. My trips to the florist, as would be expected, in the past included many bouquets for sick friends that I held as I gently knocked on hospital doors. Now with a different mixture of anxiety and hope I ring doorbell buzzers, check my hair, and decide if this is the date where I reveal my HIV status along with the bunch of flowers hidden behind my back.

Understanding the shifts in both of these domains has convinced me that as a society we must come to look at this virus as another hurdle many face in love and relationships and that we must realize that HIV does not prevent them from occurring.

MICHAEL MANCILLA

LOVE IN THE TIME OF HIV

INTRODUCTION

*Sex is easy. Love is not. Sex is pleasurable.
Love is . . . well, a bit more complicated.*

R elationships are hard work, as any trip to the self-help section
of your local bookstore will attest. Throwing HIV into the mix
invariably makes relationships even harder—disclosing HIV status, negotiating safer sex, committing to another against a land-
scape of uncertainty. All of this and more can be overwhelming and
unnervingly intrusive.

But therein lies the crux of the problem. Our worries today
arise in a whole new context. Ten, twenty years ago, dealing with the
world of AIDS only meant ugly and swift unjust deaths. Today we
have the luxury of worrying about how to date against the backdrop
of HIV. It is this new challenge that is the subject of this book.

You *can* date with HIV, as the people you'll meet in the following pages demonstrate. The virus doesn't have to mean an end to
love and romance. The question is how to traverse the inevitable
hills and valleys. We hope to answer that question in the following
chapters, offering you some new skills, some sage advice from many
who have already been there, and a little comfort. Too often gay
men have avoided closeness with other men while desiring true intimacy with them because of HIV-related fears. From sharing our status to sharing our lives together, the goal ultimately is to find and
keep love and romance with the same diligence we invest in our
health and that of our partners. We've been setting the stage for a
long time.

The Sexual Revolution, Stonewall, and Love American Style

The year 1969 saw the end of the era of "Free Love in America" and simultaneously, in June, the death of Judy Garland, a gay icon. This sparked the emotional fuel that within hours "flamed" into the Stonewall riots. It began when a gay bar in New York City was raided and some drag queens decided to fight back, an event often referred to as the start of gay civil rights.

The 1970s became a period for many gay men to begin to both explore and celebrate their sexuality. New ideas of coupling abounded. The rage was *Love American Style* on TV, which looked at how we dated and expressed our sexuality. What we did after sex was not limited to the options of marriage or sex without commitment. For many, the growing trend was "shacking up," or living together. Gays and lesbians were locked out of one option, marriage, and though many fulfilled society's expectation by becoming "mod swingers," there existed another way on this pendulum of passion: those who pushed against this trend and did couple (see the box).

Is HIV Our Vietnam?

Another social phenomenon factored into the creation and foundation of who was coupling with whom. The war in Vietnam brought back many young veterans who were physically and emotionally disabled. Some had left young brides behind at home. Some were returning to girlfriends who were expecting to pick up their lives where the war had intercepted them: with marriage and children and a future together. Suddenly, the disabled were among us in force, and they were loving and having relationships just like everyone else.

As a result of and parallel to this turn of events, a movement was born to socially integrate those who are differently abled into the mainstream of society. During the past 30 years legislation and a concurrent shift in attitude has allowed the differently abled, previously sequestered in institutions or cared for at home, to go to school and to work and to have the full spectrum of social relations.

As the nation watched young men and women returning from

SEX WITH LOVE VERSUS SEX WITHOUT LOVE

Loving sexual relationships

1. Advantages
   a. Emotional satisfaction, security, and expectation that the relationship will endure when sexual desire and passion diminish.
2. Disadvantages
   a. Some may find emotional involvement to be inhibiting to sexual expression.
   b. Confusing lust with love can generate an endless amount of resentment and bitterness.

Loveless sexual relationship

1. Advantages
   a. Feeling more free to express oneself sexually and experiment in this arrangement, gaining greater sexual satisfaction.
2. Disadvantages
   a. Sex not founded on love has a tendency to become quickly stale, dull, and boring.

Vietnam, whether the disabled veterans were spat on or welcomed would have subtle psychological ripples affecting how we respond today to those who return home from the clinic with their positive HIV test results. This acquisition of values and beliefs would help shape the response to a generation of young men (and some women) who would face either stigma and shame or reintegration into the family and society. It would certainly help determine whether the HIV positive would be welcomed into and allowed to have romantic lives.

The movie *Forrest Gump* told the story of a boy in braces breaking free (as he runs from school bullies in a field) of one physical disability and how the world around him struggles with his other perceived disabilities, to which Forrest retorts, "Stupid is as stupid does." All the while he maintains his love of his blond-haired, blue-eyed childhood sweetheart who has her own invisible afflictions—childhood abuse, addiction, promiscuity—and dies young of an "unexplained and mysterious illness" (and, since the movie is set in the 1980s, you figure it out).

At Forrest's wedding, we meet again his commander in the war, who may be missing his legs but not the capacity and right to love as he is escorted by his beautiful Asian fiancée, who is not disabled. These messages, as well as the undeniably lovable way Tom Hanks plays the role, further built the precedent for our understanding of the struggles and joys of people living romantically after the greatest challenge of that generation, Vietnam, as we do the same with our own generation's challenge of HIV/AIDS. I would offer, as does Forrest, who perhaps has survived both Vietnam and AIDS, that "Life [can be] like a box of chocolates."

Luke, HIV positive and in his twenties, like Forrest, wants to be considered human and not a virus: "Sometimes you just get really tired of being treated like a germ; you know, some people make you feel like you're just a disease. They forget you're a human being." As human beings, gay men have the right to enduring relationships, and especially since the 1960s and '70s, when cohabitation became acceptable, they have shown the inclination to pursue them, regardless of HIV status. In this book we show many of these men grappling with the challenges of HIV in their intimate lives, reaping the value of enhanced intimacy with all of its accompanying benefits. You can have this human right if you choose to exercise it.

Beyond Safer Sex

Although the AIDS crisis has left its teenage years and should be moving beyond its exclusive preoccupation with sex, as a teenager might well do when entering adulthood, the public emphasis when discussing HIV is still whom to have sex with, whom to avoid, safer sex, unprotected sex, abstinence from sex . . . and so on. Public educational campaigns still resemble an eighth-grade health teacher's admonitions about the "exchange of bodily fluids" or conversely appeal only to the libido, declaring that "Safe Sex is Hot Sex!"

To learn and teach others about safer sex, the public has had to get used to a once-taboo vocabulary: latex, water-based lubricant, blow job versus hand job, condoms, anal intercourse, dental dams, oral sex, vaginal intercourse, and masturbation. We know the dirty words that can keep us alive (and get surgeon generals fired, as when Jocelyn Elders discussed masturbation). Granted, this knowledge is a good thing. HIV can be a life-and-death situation, and sex with HIV-positive people can now be "safer" while not risk free.

No one, however, has bothered to make romance and love any less risky for people with HIV.

Regardless of one's serostatus, love is a tricky business. While there may be some universal precautions for the bloodstream, there are none for affairs of the heart. Vulnerabilities, old guilt trips from parents, cold feet, the toilet seat left up, and commitment are hurdles enough for most. In fact, the bread and butter of the counseling profession is relationships—trying to find one, maintaining one, or ending one. In this book we acknowledge that working with HIV-positive clients has added another dimension to the field.

Every day a new group of people are diagnosed with HIV. Hearing the words I heard—"I'm sorry, it came back positive"—is one of the most transformative and emotionally charged moments in life. The shock of a new identity burns through the flesh, charring the spirit and scorching the soul. In response, some feel branded, like Hawthorne's adulteress, with a modern-day scarlet letter: "This person has violated a sexual taboo."

Those of us with the virus are well aware of the stigma we are carrying. In place of "I was diagnosed with the AIDS virus" or "I am HIV positive," many of us find ourselves saying "I'm HIV." This construction of identity around a disease is unique in its personal and social ramifications. We do not say "I am the flu" or "I am breast cancer" or even "I am syphilis." With "I am HIV," an individual implies that "I am this virus and a pariah in this society; this is my scarlet letter." When someone who "is" HIV starts to date, or romance a potential mate, this identity, this stigma, often comes along for the ride.

As a community, gay men were the first to move beyond the questions of safer sex and begin to ask the more difficult questions: "Can I fall in love with someone who is HIV positive?" and "Can I fall in love *as* someone who is HIV positive?" We've seen this acted out on the stage, in fiction, and on the big screen, but for many these questions are still unanswered—yet to be played out in their own romantic lives.

It's not "I'm HIV positive" or "I've been diagnosed with the AIDS virus" anymore, but "I'm HIV"—a powerful acknowledgment that HIV carries a stigma more weighty than any other disease today.

The Interviews

There are, of course, many people with HIV who are well adjusted and living out their lives quietly and productively. This book is intended to show only one aspect of the lives of gay couples and single gay men: how we experience the impact of HIV on intimate relationships, from brief encounters to lasting love. The advice, comfort, and skills that we pass on in this book come from real people whom we met in a variety of settings—in therapy sessions, community groups, and their own homes. While some of them were already seeking help for problems related to their HIV status, many were not.

We interviewed mostly those living in an urban setting, though the personal stories of the people in this book came from a cross section of gay men who were single, coupled, or even tripled, who were just finding out about their status and not certain if they would be dating anytime soon, or, like me, had known their status for a while, may have lost a lover, and were beginning the process all over again.

Many men seemed open, even eager, to be interviewed once they knew that I too was HIV positive. In fact, many of the men we interviewed expressed a willingness to have their identities revealed in this book that is surprising only if one is unaware of the culture of sexual ethics and altruism that has arisen in the HIV-positive gay community. Our interviewees knew, as we did, that authenticity and candor were critical to relaying a credible message about the right of the HIV positive to have love—and, yes, sex—and the obligation to practice the safest sex possible and disclose HIV status to all sexual partners. Therefore we have made painstaking efforts to preserve the essence of all anecdotes and interviews while choosing to protect the identity of those generous enough to share their experiences with us and our readers.

While this sample is not strictly representative of the entire public living with HIV or those affected by it in their intimate lives, we tried to capture a broad range of personalities and situations and to represent an authentic diversity of experiences and views. This means we have included anecdotes and interviews about unsafe sex practices that we don't advocate but that still occur today, in the gay community and elsewhere, for a host of psychological reasons. We'll explore those reasons on the way to achieving this book's goal: to suggest alternatives by which all gay men can have the fulfilling sex and love lives they deserve despite HIV. To complement our own views on this complex and challenging topic, we also reference other experts' research on specific topics within this field throughout the book.

Though HIV has hit the straight community along with the gay community, there are aspects of gay culture and customs that make dating and mating different for us, and many of the issues we face simply don't apply to heterosexuals. For that reason, this book addresses HIV, romance, and sex only for gay men. As a clinical social worker who has worked with a variety of couples and individuals, however, I am struck by how many of the issues discussed here arise for those of every sexual orientation. HIV affects us all.

How This Book Is Organized

The book is divided into seven chapters, roughly following the chronology of gay male relationships. All too often it comes up later rather than sooner, but disclosure is the first thing that any man, HIV positive or negative, should think about when anticipating a sexual encounter or the beginning of a relationship. That's why it's the subject of Chapter 1, which attempts to answer the tough question of when and how you should reveal your HIV antibody status. There's no question that disclosure is a moral obligation, but in some states it is a legal obligation as well.

For many men positive status throws them into crisis, immobilizing them and plummeting them into depression; for others it has the opposite effect, motivating them to improve and transform their lives. Chapter 2 relates the ways in which many men have turned their HIV crisis into an opportunity for growth, not just in love but in every aspect of life.

How does serostatus affect your choice of sexual partners and life partners? Chapters 3–5 explore the variable and rich ways HIV factors into relationships, both short and long term. How we treat the risk of disease transmission, the hopes we craft and the fears we harbor about the future, how we communicate with one another, how we arrange our sexual lives, and other issues are considered for serodiscordant or "mixed-status couples," positives with positives, and negatives with negatives.

Health matters are never too far in the background for gay men in the age of AIDs. In fact they demand so much of our attention that we often tend to neglect the health of our relationships. In Chapter 6 we look not only at how men deal with various levels of physical health but also at how to recognize a healthy relationship—and how to leave an unhealthy one.

Chapter 7 deals with the painful topic of the loss of a loved one to AIDS—an event that fortunately occurs less frequently than it used to—and what is known as "The Lazarus Syndrome," or "coming back from the dead" (prompted by current drug treatments) and how this impacts relationships.

Liz Seaton offers invaluable legal advice in Appendix A, from how to find a lawyer to your rights to marry, property rights, financial protections, and more.

Every story has an epilogue, of course, and ours leaves you with the same message with which we begin: HIV has been redefined by current drugs and treatments, and so might the emotional ramifications of a relationship with someone who is positive. Through this book, we hope you find that "positive" possibilities await you, as gay men with or without HIV, in your future romantic encounters.

ONE

TELL AND KISS
The Skill of Disclosure

The first and biggest hurdle you will encounter when you are HIV positive and dating is how people will react when they find out the news. For this reason we address the challenge of revealing your status in the first chapter. In the following pages we have given tips and outlined ways to disclose your HIV status. Real-life scenarios showcase how people like you have dealt with disclosure—their own and that of others.

Disclosure can play itself out in a variety of ways. You can share your status before you meet your date in person, such as over the Internet, or in a personal ad; after a few preliminary dates when you know you'd like to pursue the relationship further; or, the least preferred, after your date finds out on his own and consequently feels deceived and taken advantage of.

The fact that disclosure to a sexual partner is an ethical and, is some states, legal obligation doesn't change the reality that for many of us disclosing our HIV status is even scarier than asking someone out on a date. Because of rejection by family and friends, disclosing to a potential or current lover may be a paralyzing experience. People have used different ways to avoid actually saying the words "I am HIV positive" to someone they care about and would like to become intimate with—emotionally or physically. If a committed relationship is what you want, you must get there in your own time, which could mean waiting a bit before disclosure. But committed monogamous relationships are not for everyone, and we need to look at how to negotiate other options. Most of the following disclosure techniques are more or less effective, depending on what it is you are looking for romantically.

In the following scenario, Fernando negotiates multiple partners in two different cultures.

A Tale of Two Parties:
The Monthly Social and the Escándalo Club

Regardless of how much he calls himself "the ugly Latino," Fernando looks good in black. He takes time to shine his clunky army boots, which go with his faded black jeans and T-shirt. Slicked back and cut short above his ears, his inky black hair is thinning. His black moustache looks as if it bridges his face. He is not a model by any means, but his smile exudes a warmth that draws in just about anyone. He is going out tonight, and so Fernando takes his time getting ready.

Fernando stops first at the Monthly Social, an event for HIV-positive men held in Washington, DC, that actually occurs about twice a month. The crowd—mostly white professionals—is full of friendly faces. People mill around the first floor of the house, spilling out the back door into a porch and garden. Fernando settles himself in next to an old friend from these parties and begins to chat. Early in the evening the voices move in waves. Collective "seven-minute lulls" happen spontaneously as people pause to catch their mutual breath, think a minute, or come up with the ultimate pickup line. The gathering is not loud enough to annoy the neighbors, but Nirvana is blasting at the right volume to signify a real party. People shout at each other while they try to chat and flirt.

The rumble of conversation becomes intermixed with Spanish as more of Fernando's Latino friends arrive. This group congregates, disperses into smaller groups, and moves about the party. Mostly the Latinos stay together. Fernando, however, moves back and forth between his English-speaking acquaintances and Spanish-speaking friends. Conversations all over the party range from work to gossip about the HIV community to the latest Tom Cruise movie to comparing medicinal regimens. Of course, there is also the flirting.

These monthly socials are reminiscent of apartment parties hosted by gay men and lesbians during the 1920s and 1930s. Historian George Chauncey describes similar events in *Gay New York: Gender, Urban Culture, and the Making of the Gay Male World 1890–1940*, as "hosted on a reciprocal basis among friends, or on a grander scale by men of exceptional means. . . . Many such parties were small invitational affairs, but others were immense and became regular events on gay men's calendars. . . . Parties, whether held in palatial penthouses or tiny tenement flats, constituted safe space in which a distinctive gay culture was forged." At these parties lesbians and gay men could socialize, dance with, flirt with, and kiss whomever they chose with little fear of arrest or bashing.[1]

Before World War II, these and other social events had an unwritten rule of confidentiality. Their comfort and ease were contingent on no one's tattling on anyone else. Many who attended were still considered heterosexual at work and by their families. To preserve their jobs and lives, the people at these gatherings knew it was wise to keep quiet. Of course the parties could not be advertised in regular papers, so information about them spread by word of mouth. Today, like the pre-1960s parties, the Monthly Social remains a confidential and therefore safe gathering space. The continuing prejudice against people with HIV/AIDS necessitates this secrecy; it is because of this that the gathering resembles gay parties before the sexual revolution of the 1960s.

Because a different person hosts each event, there are phone and e-mail trees to let people know about them. To find the address of a party, you call a phone number or access a web page and leave your name and phone number.

The rule about confidentiality may be unwritten, but it is definitely spoken. An announcement is made at each event so there is no mistake.

The Monthly Social was inspired by a drug trial at George Washington University Hospital in the late 1980s. The drug in question had to be injected once a month intravenously. So once a month this group of HIV-positive gay men sat around a hospital room with a bag full of medicine dripping into their arms intravenously while they chatted. The drug proved ineffective, but the social gatherings that it created were not. These men decided to continue the social aspect of the gathering sans IV drips, and years later the party is still going on.

When Fernando leaves the party, he has two phone numbers from two very attractive men. One of the men even invited him home for the evening. Having plans, Fernando declined the offer. He assumes that the boys are attracted to his muscular upper body, but what is most appealing about Fernando is that he knows how to work what he's got. He is a great friend, very outgoing, and a genuinely affectionate person. When he hears that you are thinking of going to Florida on vacation, he'll call his best friend's cousin who can get great airfare deals. If you have a friend in Peru who is having trouble coming to terms with being HIV positive, give Fernando his address. He'll sends HIV-related materials written in Spanish and do all he can from his computer in Washington, DC.

Two to Tango, Three to Tell

Later that night, walking up the steps to the Escándalo—a gay Latino club and the location of the second party on his agenda—Fernando runs into friends. All races and ethnicities are represented here, and the music has a Latin beat.

Fernando is at home at the positive parties because he doesn't have to pretend to be negative. It is a relief not to have to reveal or even debate disclosing to a potential date/lover. At the Escándalo club he doesn't have that luxury, but it's comfortable for him for another reason—because he can rest his second and sometimes awkward language, English. He chats with the woman taking money at the door and doles out hugs and kisses to the people who follow him in. He has not been here in a while, but they still know him. The music thumps through the hanging speakers. TV screens, flashing images of the Latino equivalent of the Emmy Awards, hang above the bars at either end of the club. Colored lights illuminate the dancers. Sometimes the dance floor is so tight with people that you cannot dance without touching the person next to you.

Fernando weaves through the crowd to find a spot to dance. Because it is a Saturday—drag show night—there are hordes of attractive people here, checking themselves and each other in the mirrors lining the halls. Some come early so they will get a good spot for the show. Others come early so they can dance before it gets too crowded. Still others arrive in droves just before the drag show. He looks for a spot out of the speakers' line of fire, deep in the waves of dancers. This club is a gold mine and a minefield all in one. Even before HIV status comes into the picture, rejection and acceptance lie behind every smile and within every sway of a hip. But for now Fernando just dances and looks sexy. If he gets a number here, he will have to think about when and how he will reveal his status.

When the beat flips into merengue, couples begin to hold each other as they dance. Here they can dance the moves they grew up with—merengue, salsa, rhumba—while holding the person they love or would like to love in their arms. Men twirl men, and women twirl women. Every so often, an impromptu dance lesson is had on the floor, but for the most part the amateurs make a little room for the experts. When it is finally time for the drag show, people are dancing so tightly that it is impossible not to touch your neighbors. The sweat flows.

The Fear of Telling

"I am a very bad boy," says Fernando as he begins his story about why he has three boyfriends. He fills his story with a running commentary of self-inflicted moral judgments. Because he thinks himself unattractive, he allows himself to be seduced by beautiful words from beautiful men. Of his three boyfriends (and the occasional weekend visitor), only one knows that he is HIV positive.

Fernando's fear of disclosure comes from experience. More than once a potential lover has hugged and kissed him, saying "It's all right, we can still be friends." Then they never call back. Fernando has quite a few friends, and he certainly doesn't need friends who do not call back, so he fears putting himself in a situation where he can be hurt like that again.

Fernando also likes having three boyfriends, and he's afraid that if he tells his boyfriends about his status they will leave him. His fear is, of course, complicated by the fact that he has known the three men for a while and still has not told two of them. Every day that he does not disclose his status, his fear of rejection doubles and triples; he hears in his head the surprise and shock: "What!?! Why didn't you tell me earlier?" The longer he keeps it a secret, the harder it is to break the silence.

Withholding disclosure and having multiple partners could also be ways for him to ward off commitment at this time in his life. He is doing so much (his work, school, volunteering, and socializing), he claims, that he does not have time for a long-term relationship. He does not want to be tied down. Yet, he believes, if he discloses his status, one of them might start to worry about him, and that would make him feel as if he had to get serious about that relationship.

For now, Fernando dances. He flirts with an older white man in the crowd. The older man keeps his eyes on Fernando, but Fernando pretends to ignore him. He continues to dance, making sure that he is in the sight lines of the older man. Whenever he leaves the dance floor, he is sure to brush past this man whom he is intent on ignoring. Because of family obligations the next day, he is going home alone tonight. Therefore, he can flirt without the immediate fear of rejection or disclosure.

Flirtation to Penetration: When Does He Need to Know?

It's not always that way, of course. Every flirtation that could end in emotional or physical intimacy brings a decision point: to tell or not to tell. It's easy to understand why Fernando and many others find disclosure difficult, even though failure to disclose denies their partners the right to make their own decision. Some men simply cannot face this decision point, especially when they'll have to do so over and over. So they navigate the issue in a variety of ways.

Celibacy

Clubs urging chastity vows for teenagers have sprung up across the country. Women have begun reclaiming not only their bodies but their hymens as well and proclaiming themselves "born-again virgins." These movements have gained some momentum (and federal funding) across America, but abstinence-only messages targeting gay men have not gathered much steam. However, celibacy even temporarily, is one choice that some men make, though not always just to avoid disclosing their HIV status. "Sex is how I got the disease," one man stated. "I have to heal first—you know, emotionally." Some of us who are recovering from sexual abuse or bad relationships also need this time for healing (see the box). While celibacy limits physical intimacy, it can expand the limits of emotional and spiritual intimacy.

At times, of course, celibacy does grow out of the fear of rejection. Those of us who have been rejected by family and friends because of our status can find revealing our status on a date downright impossible to deal with emotionally. Furthermore, many of us are surprised to find out that an HIV-negative person would date us regardless of our serostatus. As we learn more about the disease and meet

> Surprisingly, a national study that looked at the prevalence of celibacy among gay men found that 24 percent of us are living sex-free lives, which is twice the rate of our straight male counterparts.[2]

more people who are dating and romancing us, we can begin to allow the experience of expression of sexuality back into our lives.

Celibacy can also grow out of the newly diagnosed person's fear of infecting or reinfecting a partner. The latex condom may have become an even thinner barrier since you became positive. I have fretted over the possibility of infecting my partners and wonder who will be blamed if any of my partners seroconvert—the condom manufacturer or me. Navigating this question is part and parcel of how we decide to express intimacy in honest and aware ways.

Anonymous Sex

Some choose to avoid emotional intimacy and its incumbent risks by having anonymous or casual sex because they do not feel the need to disclose their status in those situations. While those interviewed for this book emphasized the importance of letting your partner know about your HIV status, many of them emphasized a difference between anonymous or casual sex and a really serious relationship. They also stressed the different obligations to disclose their status in these two situations. In back rooms, parks, and other places used for public sex, a "buyer beware" standard has come into play. The assumption is that any individual entering a place for anonymous sex knows the risks involved. Therefore, the unspoken rules say, as long as safer sex is practiced, a positive individual is not required to tell the partner of the moment. The rules change if you are actually dating someone and having a real relationship with him. Most of the men in my practice insist that partners should know. Not all, however, have followed through on this. These men alternate between dating with disclosure and anonymous ejaculation in silence, despite the obvious ethical problems with the latter. More so, it often comes down to intent, whether the goal is to hook up or perhaps get more serious and maybe have a long-term relationship. Hence the incidence and proportion of not only guilt and shame but hopes for acceptance directly correlate to how long and well they know their partner and the intent of the sexual encounter.

The Keogh and Beardsell paper (see the box) illustrates an unexpected "disclosure disincentive" as well. Of the respondents who reported a dramatic increase in sexual activity and number of sexual partners, most reported increased anxiety over disclosing their status. The respondents were more worried about an invasion of privacy than they were about rejection, especially if they were looking for casual sex. Some of their sexual partners became overly interested in their health and their life outside the casual sexual encounter, and the respondents saw this "as an invasion of privacy or as simply distressing." In other words, the respondents were looking for sex and felt it their duty to tell their partners about their status. However, when the partners started asking questions about health or bereavement, the respondents were offended. To avoid such encounters, some stopped disclosing to their casual and anonymous partners.

The above report continued: "Respondents reported being in a double bind if they disclosed their HIV status.

"SEXUAL HEALTH OF HIV-POSITIVE GAY MEN"

In a paper presented by Peter G. Keogh and Susan Beardsell at the 11th International Conference on AIDS in Vancouver, the sexual activity of newly diagnosed men was examined. Directly after diagnosis, some men dramatically increased the numbers of men they slept with, while others decreased the number of their partners. The men who increased their sexual partners "reported a preference for having no emotional or social connection with their partners." Having little to no connection to our sexual partners makes it easier, and sometimes preferable, not to disclose our status.[3]

They risked negative or inappropriate reactions which make sexual encounters prohibitive. If they did not disclose, they risked being 'found out,' or having to disclose after they had perhaps risked infecting a partner."[4] This double bind is even more complicated if the anonymous encounter results in an ongoing relationship. It is this double-edged sword of disclosure that makes anonymous sex so attractive and dangerous at the same time.

Regardless of the occasional crackdown against bathhouses, back rooms, sex clubs, and the like, there has been a gradual rebirth of this culture of public sex since the mid-1990s. Established venues for public sex allow gay men a place for anonymous and casual encounters without the threat of homophobic attacks. The sexual atmosphere—whether or not safer sex is encouraged—mainly reflects the attitudes of the host or owner of the establishment. Gay men, and others who have been affected directly by the HIV epidemic, are more likely to encourage safe sex by providing condoms and lubricants. This community often monitors itself. Many of the participants at jack-off parties or in establishments where safer sex is the norm will intervene when someone tries to engage in unsafe sex. Those who attend the safer-sex parties are, for the most part, people who are dedicated to safer sex. They are less likely to engage in unsafe sex even when it is offered to them.

Socials and the Personals

Somewhere between celibacy and anonymous sex with strangers lies a place where you can meet people who already know your status. Depending on where you live, this may take a little more work, but if you really want to find people you can relate to and can accept your status, it is worth it. There are social organizations like the Monthly Social, created primarily for singles, that Fernando attends. You can also find people over the Internet or by placing personal ads that announce your status in advance, which eliminates the necessity for disclosure altogether. The Monthly Social is not the only one of its kind, but it is an interesting model that could be replicated in other cities and for other communities like heterosexuals (see the box on the next page).

David, the man in charge of organizing the socials, would like to see them grow so all people affected by HIV would feel comfortable coming to the parties, but the social regulars seem to like to

For more information on this group and links to other parties/socials around the country that provide a safe, casual place for positive people to meet, visit their webpage at *www.hopedc.org.*

know whom they are talking to. On the occasions when a "married" or negative man attends the party, David will invariably get a few complaints of "I spent 20 minutes talking to him, only to find out he was negative." By having only positive, available men at the parties, David assures the partygoers of several things. First, that they can avoid the awkwardness of disclosure: we do not have to find the right words because everyone at the party is hitting for the same team. Second, that the "undesirables"—in this case, among men who date only other positives, the HIV-negative men—have been weeded out. Most important, these parties provide a space for camaraderie. At least a couple times a month, there is a place to gather and be where no one has to explain his HIV status or sexuality. With all of that gotten out of the way, the partygoers can get down to the important question: Who are you?

WANTED: YOUNG MAN, SINGLE AND FREE

Personal ads present a space where we can announce ourselves as available, attractive, and either positive ourselves or willing to date someone who is. As I stated in my introduction, I met quite a few interesting people, both positive and negative, through a personal ad that clearly defined my serostatus. This precluded the need to reveal my status to anyone I might meet through the ad. Because it is likely that gay men are more used to having HIV-positive people in their social circles, they may find that more people are willing to answer their ad when they reveal their positive serostatus. Regardless, gay or straight, revealing your status will guarantee that the respondents will accept you for who you are.

Writing a personal ad is a useful exercise whether or not it is ever published. Making a physical list of your own qualities and the qualities you need or find interesting in someone else makes weeding through the throngs of potential partners a little easier. Not only does it show the world what *you* have to offer, but it also makes it easier for others to see that you may not fit *their* image of the ideal mate and they can go on reading without hurting anyone's feelings. This exercise also serves as a self-esteem booster as you get to list all your sexy, lovable qualities while helping you crystallize (in your own mind) what you're really looking for. This may also help you realize you're ready for long-term relationships, dating, or just making new friends. Too often we as gay men have been accused of being overly obsessed with physical attributes to the detriment of accepting potential partners as whole people. In reality the way we want to be treated is not to be unduly accepted or rejected because of our HIV status.

Because most venues want you to pay for the ad by the word, you may want to be sincere, witty, and clever while getting your point across in very few words. So you must prioritize the points you want to make about yourself and about the relationship you are seeking. If you decide to run the ad, let a friend or two read it first (make them promise not to snicker) so you can make sure that you are saying what you mean to say.

If we wrote personal ads that listed what we want in a man and a relationship, the only requirement we would all have in common would be to be accepted or rejected on the basis of something other than our HIV status.

There are other venues besides newspapers in which to place personal advertisements. Many magazines have a section devoted to personal ads. Many of them have a specific slant such as vegetarian, Christian, or "alternative lifestyles." You can even post personals on the internet. Two excellent websites that specialize in positive personals are *www.positivepersonals.com* and *www.livingpositive.com*. Both allow you to do geographic searches by state or internationally, as well as view pictures and profiles of other positive individuals looking to connect.

Four before You Score:
A Model for Dating and Disclosing

Unfortunately, places like loud gay bars or other gay venues may lend themselves to physical intimacy first and something more meaningful only later. Being on a crowded dance floor or in the audience of a drag show doesn't leave much room for talking, which is necessary if you are to reveal your status. One challenge to overcome is the rapidness with which many people—gay and straight—go from first meeting to genital contact. Many gay men that I have talked to over the years have described meeting someone, having sex, maybe getting a phone number, and then never hearing from the other man again. Repeating this cycle may provide opportunities for sex but not for the intimacy that engenders trust, creates closeness, and nourishes the souls of both parties involved.

A bar magazine I ran across in San Francisco highlighted an old dating model (developed by Dominic Capello, a writer and media designer) with a sexy new name: "Score on Four." This model, which I borrow from and elaborate below, encourages getting to know a person as a human being through four dates. This will give you enough time to figure out if you really do want to sleep together, while providing a comfortable space to reveal your status to each other. If things are going right, this time will build sexual tension so that, when you finally get around to "scoring," the quality of the sex should reflect time well spent.

We as HIV-positive people are expected to reveal personal information about ourselves very early in a relationship. Without the HIV factor we were allowed to take our time building trust within our relationships. The revelation of such personal data forces you to make a leap into trust that you may not be completely comfortable with. Then again, your disclosure can pave the way for an honest dialogue about the physical aspects of sex and the emotional aspects of relationships. If you take it relatively slowly, over four dates as described below, the leap may not seem so big after all.

- *The first date:* Meet for coffee or in a place where you can talk and get to know your potential new love. Plan it to be a relatively short period of time, perhaps only one or two hours. Arrive and leave of your own volition. If you so are so moved, a kiss good night may be in order. If you want your kiss good night to lead to other things, save it for later. The point of this first date is to get to know this other person and allow him to get to know you. Flirt and gossip, but let your emotional guard down a little so the two of you can connect if possible. If you can find a place in the conversation, you can interject your status, though disclosing this early is very much up to your own discretion and willingness to confront this risk.

- *The second date:* Plan a more traditional date such as dinner and a movie or maybe dancing. It is important to have some time for conversation but also some time for the building of desire. Sitting in the dark at the movies, not really sure where his hand is, rubbing elbows occasionally, feeling your leg inches or centimeters away from his, questioning whether or not you should reach over and touch his hand—all of these can be great (if sometimes excruciating) fun. The sexuality of dancing together is understood, especially if you go to a place that encourages couple dancing as opposed to mass gyrating. If you go out for a little bite after the movie or dancing, that may be a more comfortable setting for revealing your status than during a romantic dinner or on the dance floor.
- *The third date:* Find a time and a place where the two of you can spend the day together. Go for a walk in the countryside. Visit a museum. Brunch at a retro diner or go antiquing. Spend some time together where you do not have to talk. Here you are building a nonverbal as well as verbal form of communication. These quiet times allow for a certain amount of trust. Also, this full day together helps to build a history for your relationship. If you have not already done so, you may feel comfortable enough with your new love interest to reveal your status at some point during this day.
- *The fourth date:* You may find that you have enjoyed taking it slowly with this person and thus continue on this course. After spending an entire day together, you may have decided that you do not like his politics or the fact that he matches his socks to his shirt, or whatever, and don't wish to pursue the relationship romantically. On the other hand, the two of you may not be able to keep your hands off each other (at this point making all of your single friends ill, no doubt). Unfortunately, if you have not already told your new love about your status, this may be an awkward time to do it. Springing the news about your HIV status after a sloppy, passionate kiss may surprise your date, but telling him after you have had sex will surprise him even more, with possibly disastrous results.

Obviously you can vary the scenario as you like. The idea is to allow yourself time to talk about yourselves and to disclose your status before you are on your way to the bedroom. This time for conversation during which you share your status allows your date a better chance to get to know you and time to decide whether or not your status bothers him. If the information is sprung on him directly before or after sex, the surprise itself may provoke a possible rejection more than your actual status would. Dates two and three give you time physically next to this person where a form of communication other than verbal can begin. These nudges, pokes, and playful jabs combined with open and honest conversation are the building blocks of an emotional intimacy that leads to physical intimacy, and they may make revealing your status easier.

How Do You Tell a New Partner?

When disclosing your status, think about how you would like to have the information presented to you—early in the dating process, say over coffee; while walking in the park; or in a bedroom after a long passionate kiss? Like nothing else that you could bring up during a conversation, revealing your HIV status is going to force a decision on the part of your date. By bringing up your status early in the relationship, you give your date time to consider both the emotional and health risks he is willing to take (see the box).

BETTER TO TELL: HERE'S WHY

In a study by researcher Daniel Schnell and colleagues, "Men's Disclosure of HIV Test Results to Male Primary Sex Partners," an overwhelming majority (82 percent) of the HIV-positive men who revealed their status to their partner "reported that the relationship remained 'as strong as ever' after six months." On the other hand, "most of the men who did not reveal their test results to their main partner reported being 'single' after six months."[5]

David Nimmons, author of *The Soul Beneath the Skin: The Unseen Hearts and Habits of Gay Men*, considers disclosure one of several "patterns of sexual caretaking" that include safer sex and that he sees as a form of "altruism" we engage in more than our straight peers. In his examination of the studies on which the book is based, he suggests "clearly that HIV-positive gay men tended to reduce risk behavior *more* than negative men or those unaware of their HIV status, especially with partners of different HIV status." He concludes, "It is clear that disclosure is at least in part an act of sexual ethics. Despite concerns over potential rejection, it has become a common cultural habit to disclose."[6]

Sharing your status early in a relationship instills a confidence that can facilitate intimacy, or at the very least a belief that you are an honest person. In a dating universe full of lies and head games, honesty is a very attractive quality. The honesty points you gain by disclosing early on may or may not move you from the coffee shop to the bedroom, but it may encourage a prospective partner at least to keep calling when he said he would.

> **In a dating universe full of lies and head games, honesty is a very attractive quality—maybe not attractive enough to move you from the coffee shop to the bedroom, but at least compelling enough to make him call you again when he said he would.**

Disclosure versus Revealing: A Different Mind-set

Within the HIV/AIDS community, to disclose one's serostatus has taken on a very specific connotation. Such a revelation lets someone know about your HIV status with the purpose of alerting him to the risk of contracting the virus from you. Interestingly, "coming out" as HIV positive means something a little different. We come out to our families, friends, coworkers, and even sometimes society at large, meaning we declare our status rather than hide it, not to protect them but just to be open with them. Another reason the phrase "coming out" is often used when revealing one's HIV status is that coming out with one's disease often directly follows or precedes an HIV-positive gay man's coming out as gay to family and friends.

The term *disclosure,* on the other hand, is connected to early attempts at imposing "disclosure" laws—laws designed to make it illegal not to tell a sexual partner of one's HIV status. No wonder the idea of disclosure seems so onerous.

If *disclosing* sounds like a prohibitively weighty concept to you, I suggest you think of it as *revealing* instead. Rather than disclosing the secret of your positive status, reveal it—as you would reveal anything that you felt your partner should know. Instead of positioning this act as a legal obligation, view it as an act of consideration and respect. Because his back has been giving him trouble, Fernando talks freely about the brace and how awkward it is to wear it. By not bringing it up directly, he has casually let the people around him know that he had severe scoliosis as a child and as a result wears a back brace. Because HIV and AIDS will ultimately complicate not only our lives but also the life of our date, the subject should be approached less casually.

Another way to look at this communication is as sharing. When you reveal your HIV status, you are not only broaching a subject that has health implications for your partner, you are inviting him into another part of your world. In other words, if you begin to date this person on a regular basis, you will want to share the events of your daily life. HIV and AIDS are or will be a part of that. It is painful to have a romantic partner with whom you cannot talk about this part of your life. Sharing this can be a way of opening up, not disclosing a dark secret.

Sharing and *revealing* have much more positive connotations than *disclosing*. This may seem like mere semantics, but by framing the words "I am HIV positive" differently in your own mind, you will also change the context for the person you are speaking to. I realize that for those of us who have been repeatedly rejected by friends, family, and lovers alike, changing the exact words will not change the minds of many in our lives or break down the barrier that repeated rejection has built. If you have been repeatedly rejected because of your status, I suggest continuing, for now, to socialize in exclusively HIV-positive and positive-friendly circles.

Otherwise, changing the context can have significant effects on the type of relationship you begin to form with a partner right from the start. Lee, for example, has taken an approach to revealing his HIV status that invites discussion rather than censure. Instead of broaching the subject as "Look, there is something important I have to tell you before we go on," a phrase that instills fear in the hearts of many, he begins,"I am assuming that you are positive, and you should assume that I am positive as well—does that bother you?" This particular approach opens the door to discussion. It is asking the potential dates for an opinion on which they will be judged. This way, Lee reveals his status while not allowing his prospective dates an opening to walk over him on the way to the door. "Does that bother you?" questions the assumptions of the potential date. It is a way for Lee to screen his dates as much as the other way around. It becomes a test question. If the potential date wants to continue dating Lee, he had better come up with a good answer.

Lee's approach taps into our internal list—that list of certain qualities we want in a romantic partner. We may not write the list down (unless of course you have just written yourself a personal ad), but we often have a mental picture of the ideal. We now want someone open to dating an HIV-positive person, namely, us. This may seem like an obvious requirement, but mentally adding it to our list allows us to consciously make decisions about whom we want to date, instead of settling for the first person willing to date us. By adding this new requirement to our list, we are also making sure that it is just one requirement. In other words, if he wants to date you but continually votes for Trent Lott while you usually vote for a liberal Democrat, you might want to reconsider the relationship. If this person is willing to date you but is abusive, you definitely want to reconsider the relationship. In other words, make sure you are not compromising your own well-being just to have a relationship. This dynamic of abuse is an issue we examine in more depth later in this book.

Saying "I'm assuming you're positive and you should assume that I'm positive too—does that bother you?" challenges your date to meet *your* standards and prevents him from walking over you on the way to the door.

Heroic Expectations

There are many romantic options for the HIV-positive community. However, some of us who are positive feel that we face only three romantic possibilities: expect a hero, settle for less, or do without. Several factors play into why people limit themselves to these three options. Acceptance of the stigma surrounding the disease and the assumption that a diagnosis of HIV or the onset of AIDS is a death sentence to be enacted within two to five years requires a hero in a partner. Since the disease is sexually transmitted, there's a belief that we positive people either would not or should not want to be physically intimate with anyone.

Questions crowd our heads before we disclose our status to a potential lover: "Should I tell him before we kiss?" "Will he dump me?" "If I tell him I am positive, does that mean we are going steady?" Sometimes our imagination takes us further into the future than these questions do. If you are the kind of person who picks out the floral arrangements for your commitment ceremony while imagining what-ifs before the first date, then you may also tend to ask yourself if this person will be able to be a "last love."

During the mid-1980s, a diagnosis of HIV included a two-year life expectancy. So as newly diagnosed HIV-positive people began to look for that special someone, they were looking for someone able to watch a lover die, often a heroic last love. While "first love" stories abound in clichéd literature and personal mythologies, there are no such mythologies about last loves. Only now with this pandemic disease, which attacks the young and old alike, has there been a large group of singles out there looking for a "last love." We must also keep in mind that the new drugs and treatments available are allowing some with HIV to live much longer than was previously expected.

As we learn more about the disease, as there are more and more long-term survivors, and as more and more drugs prolong our lives, our "death sentences" keep getting reprieves. Having an eight- to twenty-year (or more) reprieve, some people with HIV are second-guessing and even breaking up with their "last" loves. We really do not know how many years HIV or AIDS will take from us. And on a first date, as you sit sipping your coffee, wondering "How do I tell him my status?—will he stick around for the long run?" keep in mind that the man sitting across from you is not necessarily your last chance for love, even if you do hit it off. You may have enough time for several "this time it's for real" loves—and a few flings in between.

With the life expectancy associated with HIV having jumped from two years in the mid-1980s to as much as twenty years today, you may have time for several "last" loves—and a few flings in between.

Sometimes when we say one thing, the person at the other side of the table hears another. In other words, make sure when you tell a potential or current lover about your HIV status that he is not hearing "Are you able to care for me and watch me deteriorate?" unless that is what you really mean. Be up front and honest about your current state of health, whatever that might be. Inform him about what you are doing to care for yourself, about whether there are other people helping you out medically, and what your current support system is. This way, when you tell him about your status, you are informing him of what is going on in your life, not fishing for a nursemaid. Whether or not you imply that you are looking for a last love, your date may think that you are, so continue clearing up confusions. Emphasize to yourself and your date that this is only a date. If it were an interview for your "last love," you would have a questionnaire and a panel of friends along.

The Perfect Man

If you have created the perfect date in your head—tall, pale, and dopey; liberal, educated, and compassionate; a good cook, with a great insurance policy that includes domestic partners; some sort of medical training; looks good in a uniform—keep in mind that this picture is an ideal and probably exists only in your head. The person sitting across from you sipping coffee may be short, tan, and stocky, with some useless liberal arts degree that has nothing to do with his temp desk job (no benefits yet), who loves BBC trash sitcoms and gets squeamish watching *ER*. While he's not your ideal, this is only coffee you're sharing. Try not to worry so much about the heroic possibilities of your potential partners. Allow them the humanity that you want for yourself. People are constantly stereotyping PWAs (people with AIDS) as heroes and as superhumanly brave, when we are really only humans trying to survive our society and our disease. True bravery occurs every time we come out as gay men, practice safer sex, disclose our status, or have the courage to love and be loved.

Your potential mates may surprise you and themselves. This pandemic has transformed people in astonishing ways. We hope our friends and loved ones will grow and rise to the occasion of our lives. The people who care for people with AIDS are everyday people, doing what they need to do to care for the people they love. By trying to figure out if your date is a hero overnight, you may actually find out he is not but that his dog once chased away burglars. Either way, you get a hero in the house, even if his name is Fido and he tends to chew on the furniture.

Positive Charisma

Because many HIV-positive individuals look for partners with the same status, being positive and open about it can be a magnet for other positive suitors. The dynamic of positive–positive couples is discussed in Chapter 4, but in thinking about disclosure one must assume that some of the folk we are disclosing to may also be HIV positive. After diagnosis, we may choose only other HIV-positive people to tell about our status. Our new peers can provide empathy, support, and something that is very important when learning a new way of life: role modeling. Also they may introduce us to other venues where positive people gather, such as support groups, educational forums, and social gatherings set up for people with HIV and AIDS. New friends and support systems help to alleviate the isolation and stigma we feel postdiagnosis and before we begin dating. Also, they often cause a shift in thinking as we see people in various stages of both the physical disease and the emotional healing. By watching others continue with their ordinary lives, including participating in love and romance, we also integrate them into our lives.

Relationship Anxiety Increases Fear of Disclosure

Old fears and barriers to relationships also may be tripping you up and making you afraid of revealing your status. In other words, if you are afraid of commitment, revealing your status can be a symbol of a relationship getting serious. If you have a fear of rejection and do not feel deserving of love to begin with, you can worry about being rejected because of HIV instead of because of other, more real reasons.

While some people fear disclosing their status to a loved one, others use their HIV status to shoo away unwanted suitors. Assuming that HIV-negative people and those whose status is unknown will reject us, we might tell someone that we are positive early on just to get rid of him. Lee mentioned that he tried a few times to get rid of someone he was not attracted to by telling the suitor that he was HIV positive. He tried it only a few times, though, because the unwanted suitors were often unfazed by the news and continued their pursuit. Lee then felt compelled to come up with a nice way to say, "Well, I just don't like you."

Still others have used disclosure as a way to distance themselves from a suitor they felt unworthy of because of past drug abuse, other personal history, or even their HIV status. The thinking goes, "If I tell the suitor now, he will go away." This way you will not have to deal with him breaking up with you because of your status and breaking your heart. Another man told me stories of how he continually pushed one fellow aside because he did not feel the guy would accept him as an HIV-positive man: "It was really hard at the beginning because I . . . thought [I] would never get anyone, because I was ignorant about it. But when he started pursuing me, I would just push him away." He was scared that he would be rejected because he is HIV positive. He did not want to get involved or attached. His self-esteem had also been ravaged by years of addiction to drugs and alcohol: "Finally, after about six months I just said, 'OK, OK, I'm just gonna tell him. Maybe he'll be gone,' and when I told him, he was just like 'Is that all? I'm knowledgeable about it. I know how to protect myself.' I was like blown, totally blown away."

When I Was Told: Hearing the News of Someone's HIV-Positive Status

As part of my education as a gay man, I have had drills and emergency tests for protecting myself from catching this disease. In the gay community, having a lover or sex partner come out to you as HIV positive is something of a rite of passage. It is something that I had mentally prepared myself for. Disclosure is different and sometimes easier for gay men than for the rest of the positive population. There exists either an expectation or a belief that if you are gay you are positive or will soon be, whereas this type of fatalistic thinking is not as common in the straight world. When I

think about revealing my status to someone I care about, I can recall the first time a lover disclosed his status to me. Remembering this event and/or asking others to tell you how they felt
in that situation can shed some light on what your partner is feeling.

The first time a lover came out to me as HIV positive was in
November 1989. His name was Joseph, though with his olive skin
and Mediterranean good looks he was probably equally comfortable being called Joey. He had come to Tallahassee, where I was
attending Florida State University, for some sort of protest. Regardless of the cause, he was cute enough that his cause was my
cause. Long after the protest we found ourselves in my living
room talking long into the night. Eventually, the conversation
slowed, and a moment of silence was followed by a kiss and then
the loosening of a top button. He interrupted the moment by saying "Whoa, before we go too much further, there is something I
should tell you."

The possibilities began to immediately rush through my imagination—he had a boyfriend, a kinky sexual expectation, or some
emotional hang-up. The first two on my created list I could have
handled, but as a young therapist in training I dreaded the idea
of practicing what I had just learned in couple's therapy class on
this sweet young man in my living room. I was not expecting the
words "I'm HIV positive." With those words what had previously
been an abstract "What would I do if . . . ?" and academic "The
number of potential dates infected are . . ." became reality. The
alarms and fire drills went off in my head. This was not just a
test, not a drill. This very attractive man in my living room with
sexual intentions was telling me he was HIV positive.

Not unlike the alarms and drills in grade school, I had been
prepared for this. I knew how to hide under my desk in case of a
tornado, leave the school in an orderly fashion in case of fire, and
now as a gay male therapist in training during the late 1980s, I
knew how to put on a condom and how to avoid exchanging
bodily fluids. But, unlike tornadoes and fire, which most people
would like to avoid, I wanted to get as close to this beautiful man
as I could. I had to put my beliefs and my confidence in my own
safer-sex education to the test. Which would win out? My desire
or my dread? Was "safer sex something two HIV-negative men

do," as Vito Russo once wrote, or something I could apply to to-night's encounter? My next kiss with Joseph answered the questions, and I moved on to the next button on his shirt.

In retrospect, on that night I can say with a good deal of confidence, based on our safe behavior, that Joseph did not give me the virus. My seroconversion could have happened before or after that night. But Joseph did give me an opportunity to see and experience my own reactions to disclosure.

The Yellow Light Rule: How to Hear the News

- *Check your speed.* You may react to the news that your date is positive as you would to a yellow light at a traffic light. No matter what your own status is, you can move forward to make the light, slow down, or decide this is a good time to stop—even if that stop is just a pause to go to the bathroom to check on your condom supply. It is a bad idea to be harsh, judgmental, or accusing in front of your partner, even if it's just to scold him by saying "I'm OK with the news, but you should have told me sooner." Also, telling him "I really hope we can still be friends," even if the sentiment is sincere, most likely won't sound comforting in that setting; it will be taken as a rejection. As in driving, try not to put on the brakes too suddenly, or you and your date could experience a sudden jolt. Dating and driving both entail certain risks. How you navigate them will make the ride smoother for both you and your passenger.
- *Listen and respond.* Give yourself a moment to hear the words and acknowledge to yourself any feelings you might have (especially if this is the first time you're hearing this type of news). If your status is negative, you may choose to respond along the lines of "Thanks, I always practice safer sex," or "I'm negative," or "I don't know my status." A conscientious date will use this as an additional prompt/reminder to practice safer sex.
- *Trust and respect.* When status is disclosed, treat it in the spirit of trust and respect in which it is given. Obviously, by sharing this information your partner has some level of caring for you as a potential intimate companion. As gay men, it is con-

sidered bad form to "out" someone as being gay, and the same basic rule applies to HIV status.

As a positive man, you also have to respect the boundaries and level of comfort of your negative or untested partner. Whether he decides to unbutton the next button on your shirt is up to him.

TWO

TRANSITIONS
Reflection, Resilience, and Opportunity

We humans react to crisis in many different ways, all of them designed to help each of us adapt to the stress of a trauma like being diagnosed with HIV. It's perfectly natural to want to hole up and give ourselves the comfort and care we need to adjust to the uncertainty that comes with the virus. As we experience this transition, however, many of us end up reflecting on our lives, past, present, and future. In the process, some people feel compelled to give up on any chance for love. Others find themselves reevaluating the way they live aspects of their lives, including the way they conduct their romantic relationships with others. With this chapter we hope to encourage you to use this time to reflect, to tap into your own reserves of resilience, and to consider using this diagnosis as an opportunity for positive change if and when you feel ready to do so.

As HIV-positive people some of our current relationship challenges may be due to the fact that we are indeed positive, or perhaps we are dealing with something within ourselves that has been around for years. Fear of intimacy, alcoholism, low self-esteem, and drinking milk from the carton have all contributed to the stalling or ending of various relationships. When confronted with our own mortality we are forced to look not only at the disease but also at all the other things that make us mortal. In this way HIV, though a crisis, can become an opportunity for growth if we choose to look at it and our lives with clarity and forthrightness.

The vignettes that follow in this chapter showcase opportunities for growth after an HIV diagnosis in different people's lives. How do people handle their ongoing problems once they have been diagnosed with HIV?

Drinking, Dating, and Disclosing

Asymptomatic and attractive, Tim's slim figure, sense of humor, and charm get him a lot of second glances and dates. His light brown hair is too short to actually comb through but long enough to flatten down a little. He is quick to smile and flirt but not as quick to open his heart. Tim works for a theater company, and with his height and square shoulders, he would look good onstage, yet instead he wears a suit and tie to the office. Tim is thirty-five, HIV positive, and in love for the first time.

A dozen yellow roses sit on his dark-wood dining room table. Tim had given them to his lover, Bill. Because Bill spends so much time at Tim's house, the flowers stay. The yellow roses are Tim's attempt at giving something back, but Bill—HIV negative and already having lost a lover to AIDS—is having a hard time accepting Tim's love. The flowers stay on Tim's dining room table, but Bill is moving to Texas, the result of a job transfer.

Until recently, Tim did not believe the second glances or that people really wanted to be with him: "Confidence! I never had enough to believe I could do whatever I set my mind to do. I knew I acted very outgoing with a zest for life. I probably even came across as a little arrogant. But behind this mask I just expected that the people I met wouldn't like me."

It was more this fear and low self-esteem than his HIV status that had prevented Tim, up until now, from falling in love or maintaining a long-term relationship. Instead of the long term, Tim went for the long distance: "I always travelled for my job," which made it easier to avoid intimacy. "I had one lover in LA and one in New York." The long distance between them allowed Tim emotional space.

When Tim was diagnosed as HIV positive, much of his life changed, including his relationships. He would soon walk through the doors of the Whitman–Walker Clinic in Washington, DC, as his first step in trying to sort out and regain control of his life.

After he was charged with driving under the influence (DUI), he realized that he had been using prescription sedatives to block the fear and shame of his sexuality and, in turn, the possibility of HIV-positive status. Because of the DUI charge, he was required to attend Narcotics Anonymous (NA) meetings. Through these meetings he met other gay men working through the same internalized homophobia. These men were talking openly about their lives and their fears. So, as a part of not only accepting but also beginning to like himself as a gay man, he felt ready to walk through the doors of a clinic for testing:

"For me HIV is completely tied up with my sexuality and my shame over it. I postponed getting tested for HIV because I was afraid. Not of dying—I had already decided I was going to die—but of being forced to deal with the stigma of the virus, the stigma of my sexuality, and revealing it to my co-workers and my family."

Wrapped up in this healing process is also falling in love. It is hard to separate therapy, getting tested, and opening one's heart to love. It is almost as if in 1993 Tim unraveled the threads that are his life and he is still weaving them back together.

Crisis: Opportunity and Change

The Chinese pictograph for crisis combines the symbols for opportunity and for change. Tim shared with us the crisis of having been diagnosed with the antibodies for the human immunodeficiency virus, HIV. He also shared the opportunity to use this crisis to change his life, especially the way he views relationships.

The crisis of HIV is like other life-threatening diseases in that it forces us to look at the end of our life and how we intend to live the rest of it. But there are differences. The very transmission of this disease—through the exchange of bodily fluids—affects intimate relationships. In the age of HIV, condoms, latex gloves, dental dams, and plastic wrap are not the end-all and be-all of protected intimacy. Instead, negotiated safety and the fear of transmission to possible or current partners play a part in our relationships and dating rituals.

Because of the stigma that surrounds HIV, it transforms our

lives much differently than other crises like cancer or heart disease. With high blood pressure, it is probable that you work too hard or let life stress you out. With cancer, people wonder about inherited genes or the nearby nuclear plant. However, when we are diagnosed with HIV, people assume that we were infected through promiscuous behavior, drug addiction, prostitution, or homosexuality.

Even the "innocent" (hemophiliacs, the wives and children of bisexuals) are suspect and therefore subject to the same discrimination. As Susan Sontag says in *AIDS and Its Metaphors,* "To get AIDS is precisely to be revealed . . . as a member of a certain 'risk group,' a community of pariahs." And if you are a member of one of the risk groups, "the illness flushes out an identity that might have remained hidden from neighbors, job mates, family, friends."[1] Moral judgments from friends and family are a real possibility, so revealing your positive HIV status to the people who could be your support system is tricky. This shame, whether internalized or imposed by those around you, may affect your attempts at relationships.

Because of this stigma, the choice to walk through a clinic's doors and pick up the results from your HIV test is like walking up to the Tree of Knowledge and picking an apple. The knowledge of positive status is much like the knowledge of nakedness that Adam and Eve felt. It is like their awareness that they were not only naked but also shameful.

Even within the gay community there is still the prejudice that to be HIV negative is to be somehow cleaner than to be HIV positive.

Even within the gay community, which has been forced to live with the disease as their problem, there is still the prejudice that to be HIV negative is to be somehow cleaner than to be HIV positive. Personal advertisements clamor for partners who are drug and disease free, implying that those who aren't are undesirable.

Will Your Status Change Your Life?

So now we are aware of our HIV status. We must decide what we are going to do with this information. Needless to say, there are as many different reactions to a positive diagnosis as there are diagnoses. The mainstream media has given us some heroes to live up to, like Ryan White, who died at age nineteen, or the courageous attorney with AIDS that Tom Hanks portrayed in the 1993 movie *Philadelphia*. They have also given us pariahs like boxer Lamar ("Kidfire") Parks, formerly the world's number-one middleweight contender, who continued to engage in a blood sport knowing he was HIV-positive, not facing the virus like the hero we expected him to be. There are also the urban myths of HIV-positive people intentionally contaminating food, or of the wanton woman who picks up men and in the morning leaves the note "You now have AIDS" written on the mirror in lipstick. The rest of the population probably has to settle for a less dramatic, more "human" place in the history of HIV. Our life changes may be as difficult and heroic (but mostly unsung) as getting sober. We might become more politically active, as in joining ACT UP (AIDS Coalition to Unleash Power) or our local AIDS service organization. We may start working toward goals that previously had only been dreams, like getting that master's degree, buying a house, or going to Greece. For some it may even be as simple as spending more time with our loved ones and actually donating to National Public Radio. Whatever the manifestation, finding out you're positive changes your life in general and will definitely change your love life.

* * *

Tim continued with his healing process. He started to attend an NA group specifically for HIV-positive men. By walking into the group, he walked out of the closet (see the box). He describes how difficult it is to actually utter the words to strangers: "I can remember saying, 'This is hard—it's the first time I've ever told anybody.' But in that HIV-positive NA meeting I was telling strangers for the first time, and I didn't have control of who knew." Even though the whole point of NA is that no information leaves the room, Tim was frightened because in coming out to this small

> "Like those in love, patients wish to be known and understood, to change what they do not like about themselves, to alter what makes them unlovable. Through the erotic, light is shone on the deepest recesses of the psyche."
> —David Mann, *Psychotherapy: An Erotic Relationship*[2]

group of people he was essentially losing his power over who was aware of his HIV status. Potentially, any of the people at the NA meeting could go and tell someone else.

Since that moment Tim has come out to his family and coworkers as gay and HIV positive. Luckily, his family supports him, his mother being the primary worrier. He has also created a family of choice filled with gay men, his lesbian roommate, and other people with HIV. He even married an HIV-positive woman: "This way she gets free theater tickets, but of course the real reason was so she could get my health insurance. It's kind of kinky, but why not? Why shouldn't I? Fuck the system. They won't let me marry a man, so I'll give my health insurance to someone who needs it. I didn't do it just for her. I did it for me too."

The changes that Tim has made in his life were as much a healing from shame around his sexuality and dealing with a drug problem as they were about emotionally healing from HIV. Often HIV acts as both a catalyst and an honest mirror that reflects parts of ourselves that we can change, knowing that for now HIV is not one of them. It is through this healing that Tim allowed himself to fall in love and to be loved. To find love and to grow with love, we need to focus on our whole lives, not just a contagious virus.

Past Relationships' Impact on the Present

Most important for our purposes in this book, however, is how HIV may affect our relationships. If you were like me and were sexually active before the age of HIV, you probably had to change the way you have sex. Where some may challenge continued use of the term "AIDS crisis" for something that has gone on for so long, when it happens to you it is most certainly a personal crisis. This turning point may also allow you the opportunity to observe how you went about finding love before HIV and to change the way you do it with HIV. If your attempts at love weren't successful before your diagnosis, maybe this turning point can provide the impetus to identify and fix the problems and end up with new relationships that will have a better chance to be productive and satisfying.

Problematic Relationships: A Checklist

An exercise to consider: Grab a piece of paper and list the names of the people with whom you have had a significant relationship (for the purposes of this exercise, a relationship that lasted more than three months). If you have a picture or personal item to help focus your memory, gather those up as well. Write a few sentences about the overall relationship.

Consider these questions about your past relationships:

- Did most involve an equal or unequal power structure?
- Was the relationship mutually nurturing?
- Were you able to resolve conflict?
- Did physical or verbal abuse enter into this conflict?
- Did alcohol or drugs play into the scenario?
- Did you end most of the relationships?
- Did you try to hold on to this person beyond the end of your relationship?
- Was someone else involved?
- Did the two of you have an understanding/definition of monogamy, and was that honored by you?
- Was HIV status the main reason for the end of your relationship?

By answering these questions, you can begin to see patterns in your previous romantic life and to discover what changes are needed, which negative patterns are possible to change, and which you have already corrected. The exercise gives you the opportunity to make a commitment to maintain any positive changes you have made in the past and to take pride and accomplishment in the fact that some of these problems never have been part of your history nor will likely be in the future.

Drugs, Alcohol, and HIV

Drinking the swill to sweeten the pill . . .
—Pet Shop Boys, *Bilingual*

As described earlier, a DUI charge alerted Tim to the notion that something was awry in his life. Before this Tim didn't consciously view the use of drugs as a factor in his problems. Through NA, however, he was better able to get to the heart of what had begun to tear him up inside and deal with that head on. As he was able to incorporate this into his everyday life, he no longer felt the need to attend NA meetings.

Even without needles, substance abuse directly increases the chances of contracting or transmitting HIV. A study of gay male substance abusers proved that safe sex was difficult for them. The disinhibiting effect of alcohol and other drugs, combined with learned patterns of association between substance use, low self-esteem, lack of assertiveness, and perceived powerlessness, all led to unsafe sex, including unprotected anal sex. Gay men are no different from the rest of the population. In other words, when anyone adds drugs or alcohol to sex, it is much easier to forget about the condom or not to notice when the condom breaks. Furthermore, it is more difficult to refuse sex, or sex without protection, when you are under the influence (see the box). Even if you try to resist, your slurred words and limited awareness of what is going on around you places you and your partner at risk.

Alcohol is the drug of choice for most Americans. In general we are not looked down on for taking a few drinks; only if we cannot stop. If alcohol is high on your list of possible unhealthy patterns, it may be the alcohol, not the virus, that is preventing you from having a healthy relationship. If someone walks away from you in a bar, it may have been the slurring of the words "I'm HIV positive," not the statement itself, that sent him running.

If alcohol and/or drugs are involved in much of the pain around your relationships, you are not alone. In the United States, the fastest-growing subset of the HIV-positive population is no longer gay men but substance abusers; at least one in ten persons suffers from some form of dependency on addictive drugs or compulsive behaviors. Within the gay and lesbian community this number is three times as high.[3]

Like many gay men, I socialized in bars. I went to my first gay bar, a place called "Badlands" in downtown Cincinnati, on my eighteenth birthday. In Cincinnati at that time, you could drink only 3.2 percent (alcohol) beer. I saw my first drag queen, "Peaches," who was quite regal, from her shiny sequined gown to the large brandy snifter she carried.

Back then, glamour, sophistica-
tion, and the whole new world of
who I was as a young gay man
centered around gay bars and
brandy snifters. During the next
decade, considerable time was
spent dancing and drinking. My
friends were bored by the "same
tired crowd" and watching a lot

> If someone walks away from you in a bar, it may have been the slurring of the words "I'm HIV positive," not the statement itself, that sent him running.

of chemically altered (beyond estrogen and silicone) queens perform
on and off stage. Though they were bored, they were at the bar, with a
glass of something in their hands.

After my diagnosis, the bars somehow lost their appeal. I realized they were not conducive to conversation. I wanted the conversation to be heard clearly when I revealed my status. When we meet
someone, we are, of course, sizing him up through the use of questions such as "Do you have any hobbies?" and "Where do you
work?" The loud noise and occasional stumbling drunk are often intrusive to such conversations.

Adding alcohol impairs one's judgment in choosing possible
partners. Remember the pin that declared, "Everyone is beautiful at
3:00 A.M."? If your pin says, "Everyone is beautiful at 3:00 A.M. and
after a six pack of beer," and you wind up with someone the next
morning you didn't intend to be with, your problem is not HIV
alone, it is alcohol consumption. Many centers and clinics for people with HIV can help clients with HIV-positive twelve-step programs or counseling. Whether or not you are addicted to alcohol,
you need to find a way to stop beginning and/or ending your relationships with alcohol as a buffer.

Some people become positive as the result of injection drug
use or of being the sexual partner of a user. HIV-positive injection
drug users must understand the health risks involved in the injection process. The seriousness of dirty needles, abscesses, collapsed
veins, and septicemia is increased because of the increased risk of
various other infections, such as hepatitis B and C, as well as bacterial and fungal infections. We need to limit these stresses on our immune systems as much as possible. If you are unable or unwilling to
enter treatment, it is important to have access to clean needles,
whether through a needle exchange program, a pharmacy, or a physician. Methadone, a drug that helps minimize the strong cravings

for heroin, has been a valuable resource in stabilizing the health of HIV-positive heroin users, many of whom became infected because of unavailability of clean needles.

* * *

I thought one day I would just be struck sober.
—Richard, thirty, a person with AIDS

The moment of crisis brought by his diagnosis became an opportunity for change for Tim. In my work with patients I have found one of two kinds of reactions: (1) they increase their alcohol or drug use as they choose to swim deeper into the waters of denial; or (2) they make an energized and concentrated effort to recover and reconstruct their lives as positive, clean, and sober people. Finding partners or community-oriented environments that support and affirm your desire to get clean and sober is critical. While on staff with Pride Institute, a specialized psychiatric and substance abuse treatment program for gays and lesbians, I saw daily the need for this type of treatment for these clients, many of whom are living with HIV. In some cities there are specialized AA/NA (Narcotics Anonymous) meetings for gays and lesbians as well as meetings such as "Positively Sober" for people with HIV. Regardless of the treatment route you pursue, it will require hard work.

Drugs and HIV

Bruce has been HIV-positive for fourteen years and avoids relationships for fear of rejection because of his status. He was in a long-term relationship three years ago, where his partner was also positive.

He was left for someone younger.

Sitting on a beat-up couch, in the basement of a gay community center, at a casual weekly support group for HIV positives, he talks openly and slightly harshly about frequenting "glory holes," the nickname for a type of gay male anonymous sex venue: "I tell people I'm positive when I have anonymous sex; it's attempted murder otherwise. My status is one of the reasons I go there. Afterall, I'm more likely to get turned down for a relationship."

But it seems that Bruce experiences rejection for being too

honest as well. The day I sat in on his support group, he offered a matter-of-fact "kiss my ass" defense to moral objections of many in the group to his having anonymous sex when positive. He later told me he had decided not to attend the group anymore. Bruce stopped intravenous drug use when he was diagnosed as positive in the 1980s, starting taking his medicine, and changed his way of living. He's been physically stable for over a decade, except for anxiety and mood swings, which he treats with medication.

He says, "They don't like me at the community center, but I have the support system from being in recovery. I'm also happy being single for right now. My main goal is finding a cure since I'm positive."

At age forty, Bruce has little contact with his immediate family, who live in Philadelphia. "I'll call them and let them know I'm OK, but I don't give them my phone number or address. They're OK with my being gay, but they can't come to grips with my being HIV positive. I keep sending them literature on the virus, which seems to be helping. Just now is not the time to let them know where I am."

Bruce may have an addiction—to sex. He probably displayed good judgment by not relying solely on a peer-led HIV support group, because they cannot address the problem of his sexual compulsivity. He may benefit from one-on-one therapy, coupled with a support group for sexual addicts. Bruce is dealing with multiple stressors, and though he seems to have things under control (listening to him talk, one cannot helped to be drawn to his charisma and outward show of confidence and determination), my guess is that he's using compulsive sexual encounters to hide other pain and a lack of control in his life.

What makes an addict? That's a question which is not easily answered and is hotly debated in the gay community. While Bruce says he is happy staying single, it's questionable whether his anonymous compulsive sexual encounters are conducive to his well-being or that of others. He could be exposing himself and many unknown others to wild strains of HIV not inhibited by the current antiretroviral regimen and other sexually transmitted dieseases (STDs), and he is vulnerable to the emotional emptiness that numerous encounters of anonymous sex can bring. Additionally, Bruce's current sexual behavior pattern is delaying the possibility of having a supportive relationship.

Are You Using Easy Sex as a Substitution for the Real Work of Intimacy?

If you're facing a major roadblock, it's important to ask yourself whether you're in the right support group. If it is clear that the group is not meeting your needs or your needs are greater than what this group alone can offer, you might benefit from another intervention—including more intensive outpatient or inpatient treatment. Additionally, if you're concerned at all about the possibility of being sexually addicted or compulsive, we encourage you to get an assessment from a trained professional or attend a Sex Addicts Anonymous meeting to further assess your needs (see the box).

> Compulsive sexual thoughts and/or behaviors lead to increasingly serious consequences, both for the sexual addict and for others. Therefore, it is extremely important to identify the symptoms of sexual compulsivity and seek appropriate help.

Sexuality and having sex can be a normal part of life, even for those who are positive and single. We're not saying it's easy, but the key is to work on your personal issues, sometimes on your own and sometimes with a trusted confidant, and not use sex as an emotional substitution or escape. In the section that follows we consider another way in which trust—the cornerstone of intimacy—is violated. If either of these is left unaddressed, it can create a potential challenge to having a complete and satisfying relationship.

Previous Sexual Abuse

While we may be more familiar perhaps with the experiences of sexual abuse among women, it is something that profoundly affects men, gay or straight, as well. How that plays out and affects our intimate lives needs acknowledgement, support, and understanding as both a precursor and cofactor to our lives with HIV.

The comfortable large scarf Susan wraps around her shoulders is a warm brown color. On a cold drizzly January day in Washington, DC, it is cozy in her office. Today she looks like she has walked out of an international mail order catalog, with her elegant scarf, her black hair, and dangling earrings. She is slim, has long fingers, and vaguely Asian features.

Susan, who now identifies as a lesbian and has been living in Paris until recently, was first tested for HIV against the advice of her doctors. She was in a drug rehabilitation program in 1985, and her doctors worried about her. The combined facts that there were limited treatments available for substance abusers at the time and that Susan was fresh off the streets from drug addiction and prostitution, and had been raped in her past caused her doctors legitimate concern. In 1985 a positive diagnosis for HIV was a death sentence to be carried out within the next two years, and it's hard to tell someone she has got the rest of her life to lead drug free when her life may last only another six months.

Her story begins, "I was two hundred pounds as a teenager, and that's why I turned to drugs." She at first used her weight as a reason not to get close to people; then came drugs, and finally HIV. The drugs led her toward prostitution, and the prostitution led back to drugs. Because she went from a 200-pound teenage virgin into a cycle of drugs and prostitution, she had little time to develop a sense of sexuality, or rather intimacy, with anyone.

Susan describes her experience: "I certainly know what drugs and drinking are," and she knew when people wanted to have sex with her.

As Susan started to clear away the drugs and self-loathing, she still felt she was not meant to fall in love. She traded her drug addiction for fighting for her friends, organizing HIV support groups and protesting inadequate HIV/AIDS policies. Her sense of self increased as she became more successful in these struggles. Eventually, through her sober forays into the romantic world, she realized that her biggest problem in dating men was not that she needed to heal from her past—it was that she was not attracted to them.

* * *

> The taboo against talking about incest is stronger than
> the taboo against doing it.
>> —Maria Savzien, MD, as quoted in
>> *The Invisible Epidemic,* by Gina Corea[4]

The term *survivor* is used to describe not only PWAs and people living with HIV but also those of us who, like Susan, have lived through sexual abuse or assault. Because of the specific risks that prostitution creates, HIV infection rates are often perceived as higher for sex workers. Though numerous studies in the United States confirm that prostitution is not a significant factor in the spread of HIV/AIDS, many male and transgendered prostitutes face struggles similar to Susan's. One of the studies that supports the view that prostitution is not significantly linked with HIV is the Center for Disease Control and Prevention's (CDC's) 1993 HIV/AIDS Surveillance report, which said that only 123 out of 202,665 infected adult and adolescent males diagnosed since 1981 (0.04 percent) denied any risk factor except for having sex with a female prostitute.

Health problems associated with surviving childhood abuse are similar to those associated with surviving sexual assault as an adult. They include numbing the pain through substance abuse and/or reliving the trauma by staying with abusive lovers, spouses, and partners. As such, some survivors of childhood sexual abuse must also play the double survivor game. Dr. Sally Zierler, a researcher on sexual trauma, found that childhood sexual abuse in women increased the likelihood of HIV infection by 50 percent.[5]

Gina Corea, in *The Invisible Epidemic: The Story of Women and AIDS,* states, "The attacks, through abuse, on a woman's spirit, on her self-esteem, on her very capacity for developing an ego, an identity, a self, a sense of 'I am,' plow the ground for drug addiction. This, in turn, creates an environment ripe for HIV infection."[6]

Male Survivors

Men too are facing the challenge of surviving both sexual assault and HIV. Even though Corea specifically addresses the concerns of women—rape and sexual abuse—these cut through the psyches of men just as painfully and open men up to similar situations and risks. Mike Lew, a therapist who specializes in working with male incest survivors and is the author of *Victims No Longer,* states that as many as one in ten men are survivors of childhood abuse.[7] Several studies support this, specifically those by Doll et al. (1992), which found that of 1,001 adult gay and bisexual males attending STD clinics, 37 percent had been coerced or forced to have sexual contact with men before age nineteen.[8] Follow-up studies by the same team of researchers on this cohort saw a significant link between earlier sexual abuse, current depression/suicidal ideation, risky sexual behavior, and HIV-positive status (see the box).

Susan is indeed a longtime survivor. She has outlived all of the members of her original HIV-positive support group. She has been given a chance to heal from the attacks from various "Johns," as well as from harm she has done herself, and now she has fallen in love. But many with similar dilemmas are still wallowing around in the mud that is the hard and messy part of recovery. This initial, intensively emotional work may make a romantic relationship impossible for the moment.

I've known several men who were childhood victims of some trauma that continues to haunt them. Sensory reminders of the event—a sound, scent, or visual image that is associated with their sexual abuse—bring all the horror back to them.

Even when they try to move on with their lives they turn the corner to the strains of a certain song or a glimpse of certain clothing, and they are taken back to a place of terror and betrayal. Attempts at love and affection terrify them that much more. The early abuse affects how such men view their body. They do not assume the right to say no and have trouble assertively protecting and preserving the sanctity of their body. Whether or not they want to protect themselves from HIV infection, they sometimes do not have the wherewithal to insist on their safety standards.

MENTAL HEALTH PROBLEMS INCREASE GAY HIV RISK

A CDC Study of 2,881 men who have sex with men in New York City, Chicago, Los Angeles, and San Francisco found that those with "psychosocial" problems such as childhood sexual abuse, depression, multiple drug use, and partner violence had higher rates of unsafe sex and HIV infection. Men who participated in risky sex jumped from 7.1 percent of those with none of those problems to 33.3 percent for those with all four. Only 13 percent of those with none of the problems had HIV, while 25 percent of those with all four problems were HIV positive, the CDC reported.

—Fourteenth International Conference on AIDS, Barcelona, Spain, 2002

Resilience and Recovery

In my work as a therapist, I am continually surprised at people's resilience. One of the important things I have learned from working with survivors of sexual abuse is the need for recovery. All survivors need this, but as HIV-positive people, we must prevent ourselves from continuing to live the role of victim. Mike Lew defines recovery this way: "For me, it is about freedom. Recovery is the freedom to make choices in your life that aren't determined by the abuse."[9]

A Man Falls in Your Lap: Replacing the Isaac Newton Theory of Love

There are, of course, much less serious impediments to relationships. Maybe you're self-conscious about your looks, or you don't like bars, or you're not interested in anyone you meet through work, or your last blind date was a disaster. An acquaintance of mine works overnight, so he has almost given up on romance for the moment because he is not around when the rest of us meet each other.

But as the lottery advertisement says, "You can't win if you don't play!" Many do not actively pursue romance or relationships, believing the myth "When you are not looking for it, it will come" or "When it is your time, it will happen" and other such belief systems that invoke fate, astrological signs, or the will of God. By leaving fate or our romantic lives to others, we experience an overall external loss of control. In other words, if we are waiting around for others to come up and ask us to dance, we have no control over who might ask or even whether we get asked.

For gays and lesbians, this can be a particular problem as there are no specific guidelines for who approaches whom and who pays the dinner bill. As teenagers we were not taught how to date our own sex. Even in the highly masculine "leather bars," where one might think the situation would be different, the rate of men approaching men is not significantly higher than, say, at a straight or other kind of gay/lesbian club. Not just women are sitting around waiting for that perfect someone to appear and sweep them off their feet.

I call this passive approach to dating the "Isaac Newton Theory of Love" because it is as if you are just sitting under a tree waiting for love to fall into your lap, or into your heart, like Sir Isaac's apple that purportedly led to his discovery of gravity. After all, while gravity may be a potent force in the world of physics, it is not useful in the domain of love. By discarding this passive approach, you still have an opportunity to grow and adopt a new theory of love.

> **If lines of available suitors do not arrive on your doorstep every time you decide it is time to fall in love, go out and shake the tree. Try a few apples. If you do not find the right one, shake the tree again.**

How to Meet Someone Special

- *Meeting and dating the right man requires liking and accepting yourself.* Move past any guilt or shame you may have over either being gay or HIV positive. Learning to like yourself and choosing to live your life the way you want to may be different from how your friends and family want you to live. As long as you are not hurting anyone, you have the right to pursue your own good your own way.
- *Be available.* This means not listening to those voices in your head that say you're too old, too thin or fat, or no one would want someone who is HIV positive. Consider joining a club; become a member of your town's gay water polo team or bowling league. The secret to being available is being visible. The man of your dreams is not going to appear magically while you are watching another episode of *The Antiques Roadshow* on TV. Finding and meeting other gay and/or positive men requires you to go where they congregate.
- *Be bold, flirting instead of cruising.* First of all, don't say, "I'm too shy." Being shy is just another excuse not to meet someone. If you have a great smile, there is no harm in flashing it to someone or even the occasional wink. If your goal is more relationship oriented, rather than just getting laid, the secret is to make it a tad playful, sending a message you are interested in meeting him. This is a bit different from "cruising,"

which has more of a seductive pose or body language, implying you want to have sex with him.

Men who cruise in its rawest form are usually nonverbal or, at most, monosyllabic—standing against a wall, four fingers in their jeans' front pockets, with their thumbs framing what they hope will be the *object* of your attention. Flirting, while it can be nonverbal, requires revealing a bit of your personality with the intention of learning a bit about theirs. Learning about instead of objectifying each other will enable us to value other men and may well create a safer framework in which we can be valued for who we are, independent of our HIV status.

Boy Meets Boy: Plot Lines and Chat Rooms

It has been said that life offers one romantic story line: "Boy meets girl (or boy in our case), boy loses boy, and boy gets boy back." Now, computers offer a new way to start, and perhaps play out, this classic plot line.

The Internet as the digital coffee shop/bar/back room/ bathhouse provides new and often multiple dating opportunities. Nowadays, "boy often meets boy" through online chat rooms and by reading the posted profiles (which often can include a picture). We can now continuously scan the web and through "keyword searches" try to meet our own potential future mate. However, for some, the risk and fear of losing the date is so great that they do not move beyond

These are websites where positive men with modems can connect with one another.

Personal ads
  www.livingpositive.com
  www.positivepersonals.com
  www.planetout.com

Chat rooms or bulletin boards
  www.gaypoz.com
  www.aol.com
  www.gay.com

Along with specialized groups found at websites like Yahoo (*www.yahoo.com*), the latter two URLs may require you to do a keyword search before you get where you want.

I also invite to you to my web page for active updated information and to let me know about any upcoming events that may be of interest to our fellow Positive Paramours:

  www.hivandrelationships.com

the boy-meets-boy phase. Many of us, as gay men independent of status, need to overcome this fear. We need to acknowledge that getting to know someone involves an investment and risk, even after exposing our positive status. Coming to realize this even when facing potential loss can include the completion of the plot line, which can then end with "boy gets boy back," recovering your object of affection. So we should not automatically expect that we will lose boy by sharing our status.

> **Many men never go beyond "boy meets boy" for fear of getting to "boy loses boy" the minute they disclose their positive status. But getting to know someone always involves investment and risk, regardless of HIV status.**

Though modems have replaced traditional handshakes in allowing us to be socially and sexually forward at the safety of our desks, it is an encouraging sign that more and more men on both sides of the HIV spectrum are putting their status in their profiles, perhaps minimizing the potential risk of rejection while opening new doors on how we seek and acquire affection.

Positive and Assertive

If the AIDS epidemic has taught us nothing else, it has shown us the importance of examining, challenging, and rejecting passivity. Clearly, this fact is visible in not accepting the term "AIDS victim" by the media and in not being the "good patient" in our relationships with our doctors and health care providers if they are not giving us optimum care. The "UP" in "ACT UP," an activist group, means to "unleash power." When we sit around and wait for love to cross our path, our only power is that of saying yes or no—not much power. If we wait around long enough, we may end up saying yes to the next human with a pulse who asks . . . perhaps not the wisest choice.

The joy of being the one who asks is that we get to choose whom we ask. Do you want to date only HIV-positive people? Then flirt with people whom you know are HIV positive. And you need not restrict yourself to the bar scene. Do you like to read? Start flirting with bookstore clerks or join a book club. Grocery stores, rugby leagues, community theaters, drumming circles—there are social nooks and crannies everywhere, and you need not just go to bars to find a date. If you do not start looking, your date may not find you.

Searching for Mr. Right in the Wrong Town

Lee, HIV positive, has trouble finding "Mr. Right" simply because he lives in the hometown in which he grew up. Lee is the middle-America boy next door with an angled jaw, strawberry blonde hair, and a wide, inviting smile. He loves his rural community, but as a gay man wanting to find a life partner, he feels he needs to move to a more urban, more accepting universe. He says, "I just want to go somewhere where it's already OK to walk down the street hand in hand with somebody that you love."

Prior to his positive diagnosis, as Lee puts it, he "was pretty much content being a pseudo-closeted gay farmer, . . . the typical gay farmer in the Heartland, which is not very typical." He would vacation in gay meccas like San Francisco, south Florida, or Washington, DC. Then he would return home and speculate what his heterosexual neighbors might think: "Gosh, he's a really good cook, and he sings well, and he has a great set of Teflon cookware, and he dresses very well. . . . He's going to find a nice girl someday."

Because he is not in the market for a nice girl, and because the few nice boys in his area are either straight or have moved to more densely populated and more accepting locations, Lee is finding it difficult to find Mr. Right. Looking at his own mortality has made Lee wonder whether Mr. Right is not hiding somewhere else and decide that, if he is ever going to meet him, he had better move to larger pastures to the political left of middle America. Indeed, as soon as he finishes his master's degree, Lee is moving to the West coast.

What Are You Looking for in a Partner?

> One of the first things I'm going to do now that I'm dating again is laser the hair from my back.
>
> —Derrick, forty

Another way to form a better dating relationship is to simply rearrange the way we think about, and therefore go about finding, a new romantic partner. In other words, what do we look for in a partner, and what do we want out of a relationship? When immersed in singledom, we spend time charting out blueprints for the perfect mate. While we may not expect to find someone with everything on our list, we still have that ideal in mind when we start to flirt. For some, the blueprint contains plans that were drawn by someone else: the media or our family. We also tend to gauge our sexuality, or desirability, by the standards set by MTV, *Playboy, Vogue,* and Calvin Klein.

Sometimes this can get out of control. Relationships aside, not since ancient Greece has there been such an emphasis on masculine beauty. The increased interest in the male form runs parallel to the HIV epidemic. Having greater expectations of male beauty seems, in some ways, to be an attempt to distinguish between those who are healthy and those who are not. HIV-positive and -negative gym rats, especially in the gay community, now scurry about sports clubs attempting to live up to this distorted picture of health.

Commercialization followed as Madison Avenue picked up on this cult of masculinity during the late 1980s. Previously, only women's bodies were displayed as cheesecake at various profit venues. Calvin Klein advertisements that began featuring teen idol Marky Mark displayed as beefcake for profit. A nice set of abs or a fine ass was all that it took to sell millions of dollars worth of perfume. The rest of us have followed with our wallets and pocketbooks, not only toward these products but also

> **Having greater expectations of male beauty seems, in some ways, to be an attempt to distinguish between those who are healthy and those who are not.**

to the gym. Slim and trim is no longer the goal. Anorexia, while still prevalent, is no longer the "hip" body type. Now women and men will exercise at unhealthy rates. Nutritional supplements, aerobics, weight training, and a few more hours on the bike have replaced just plain starving oneself.

Big dick, nice body, impressive job, and great toys. That is what we—gay men and straight women—are supposed to look for in a man. Whether we admit to subscribing to a patriarchal culture or not, those values are left over from a time when the "man of the house" provided for the family. The toys are particularly important. If he has cool toys, just think how many he can provide you with.

Flashy cars, a nice condominium with lots of indirect lighting, a good sense of fashion—these things say not only "I am successful" but also "I can pay the rent." Men often feel pressured to look as if they have more than they do, just to attract a mate.

There are games we play to check up on people without directly asking "How much do you make?" Since most people do not bring résumés with them to bars, getting into someone's bed is a way to check out his real estate holdings, window moldings, and the designer labels on his sheets (which should ideally match those on his underwear). It is also a convenient way to check for HIV-related drugs in the medicine cabinet.

In college we ask, "What's your major?" The answer provides a clue to what your potential date may become, at least professionally. In the "real world," we ask, "So, what do you do?" When spouse hunting, we generally are not fishing for "What is your passion in life?" but rather "What is your level of education, class, and paycheck?" If you have two degrees but are currently working at Starbucks, your answer to "What do you do?" includes the two degrees and an exaggerated plan for the future.

But as HIV-positive people, if our answer is "I'm retired" and yet we are 35 years old, we can see the questioner's mental calculators starting to work. While you can try to imply that your *Fortune* 500 company was just bought out for a large sum of money, if you are gay, your potential date will probably assume that you are HIV positive.

Many of us, as HIV-positive individuals, however, have begun to reconsider the qualities that we want in a partner, as well as what we can offer him in return. Facing our own mortality causes us to reprioritize. We are placing greater value on the intangible, the emotional, the personality, and the spirit of the people we date. Ultimately, we want to find someone who is emotionally secure, able to communicate his needs, and able to respond to us when we express ourselves. Also high on the list is someone who has a good sense of humor, is a good conversationalist, and has informed opinions on a wide variety of subjects.

Many of us when faced with HIV make a conscious effort to live our lives more fully. As a by-product, we often get closer to the above criteria and end up being not such a bad catch after all—hairy backs, HIV, and all.

Tainted Love: Moving beyond Stigma

Safer-sex campaigns had a different meaning for me when I was HIV negative or when I did not know my status. Now that I'm positive, I look more closely at how the images of those infected with HIV are portrayed in the HIV prevention campaigns. These ad campaigns include "Winners always use condoms" (losers don't??!). Another ad stated, "So if you are going to have sex, play it safe and use a latex condom, every time." The ads implore that everyone use "condom sense."

These early ads, though they sought to avoid further alienation or dehumanization of HIV-positive individuals, implied that these positive people had made a "mistake." They were not "smart" and certainly didn't use "condom sense." Otherwise the HIV positive would still be like the rest of the population, trying to protect themselves from HIV. This mode of education creates a life-saving but unintentionally condescending message, while hoping to reinforce a diligence in our sexual behavior that for some is difficult to maintain. While we as gay men strive and for the most part succeed in our attempts to uphold this standard of sexual behavior, there is still the implicit accusation of our having contracted HIV as a result of a character flaw, which in the end leaves many men confronting their own feelings of shame and self-doubt.

Never Have Sex Again?

The message from society seems clear: we should never have sex again. Scott O'Hara, the late porn star of twenty-six videos and a former editor of *Steam Magazine*, wrote in *Policing Public Sex*:

> Gay men (and especially positive gay men) have been beaten into submission over the past 15 years. . . . [T]hey've been convinced that Positives never have sex (except for Gaetan Dugas and other Typhoid Marys). There is an image of the PWA: He has a gaunt face, staring eyes, stick-like limbs and no dick.[10]

Even if we look sexy, as a public service we are not supposed to have any sex.

In fact some HIV-positive men report feelings of lower sexual interest and desire and decreased energy, and so they don't have sex. As a therapist, I recognize this energy loss could be a symptom of depression. It is also an indicator of lowered testosterone levels, caused by HIV or drugs taken for HIV, which are treated quite differently (i.e., with testosterone gel or shots) than depression. We must decide with our doctors how to proceed in treating both impotency, muscle wasting, and decreased energy.

Impotency literally translates to mean, "lacking in power." If a doctor doesn't treat this problem, it could be an inadvertent attempt to control the spread of HIV via our sexual expression. Perhaps we are doing it to ourselves by not mentioning impotency or lowered sex drive to our doctors. To seek treatment, we must believe that the restoration of our sexual desires and sexual desirability is something we have a right to. It is a question of quality of life. If sexual intimacy is important to you, then getting this treatment is a necessary part of your romantic and sexual life, just as it would be to a prostate cancer patient or an older man. Current treatments may include Viagra, which is marketed to counter erectile dysfunction and to be taken before one plans to have sex, but caution needs to be exercised here. There are multiple causes of depression and of impotence, and therapy must be individualized with each patient in a responsible manner.

Someone with 750 T-cells, no viral load, and an optimistic outlook may have different expectations for a relationship than someone with an advanced case of AIDS, *but opportunities for love can exist for both. We need to find ways to make ourselves feel valued and truly deserving of love.*

Those of us living with this pesky virus need to be invested in our health and know what stage our disease is in. Also, we have to examine our health in context of what it means to be in a relationship—someone with 750 T-cells and no viral load and an optimistic outlook may have different expectations than someone with an advanced case of AIDS. Opportunities for love can exist for both. The awareness of your health and your ability to communicate this expectation to those you have a romantic interest in is paramount, even when you feel tainted.

As I've already said, being HIV positive makes us feel as if we carry a stain that all can see, like Hester Prynne's big red A in *The Scarlet Letter*. For some of us the stigma seems overwhelming, especially when we are first diagnosed. In the end, we need to find ways to make ourselves feel valued and aware that we are truly deserving of love.

Growing up as a Mexican American, I was taught by my parents to blend in with the pervasive and "desirable" Anglo community. People didn't discriminate against you; they were trying to normalize you. My last name, Mancilla, means "a spot, stain, or blemish." In high school, I looked up the meaning of my name. Underneath the definition was the sentence *Más vale mancha en la frente que mancilla en el corazón.* Translation: "It is better to have a blemish on your face than a stain on your heart." This old Spanish saying contrasts with what many of us have been taught to look for in a desirable partner and expect a partner to look for in us. We can use this old saying as a mantra to boost our self-confidence (especially if we have Kaposi's sarcoma, facial wasting, or any other outward sign of HIV/AIDS), as well as remember it when we are out there looking for potential dates.

Someone once told me this story:

> This afternoon I tried to remember my initiation into the power of being tainted. I think I was about six, and I had a friend of the same age named Stewart who lived on the next block. We were playing with our jump rope on the sidewalk. Suddenly, Stewart started glowering and walking away from me, saying "I don't want to play with you any more." I was flabbergasted. "Why?" I asked, on the verge of tears. Stewart walked back up to me. He looked at my neck and said, "Because of that!" Then he reached out and touched a small mole below my right ear. And then he ran down the sidewalk. My heart was broken, at least for a few minutes, maybe longer.
>
> Taint. I didn't know the word when I was six. But I think I felt the power of it as I sat on my lawn, holding my jump rope and rubbing the side of my neck.

Later on, perhaps a college boyfriend will kiss that very same birthmark and tell him how cute and sexy it is. As gay men, our first moments of awareness of sexual identity may have been followed by feelings of isolation. We need to implement the skills we used in overcoming that isolation by meeting others who accept us— whether we are gay, have a birthmark, or are HIV positive. Ultimately, we find that we are not alone. After all, it took someone else to make us positive.

THREE

LOVE
IN CONTRAST
Negative and Positive

D oug, who appears to be in his middle to late twenties, arrives at *POZ* magazine's Life Expo health fair, currently on tour in Washington, DC, six weeks after receiving his positive diagnosis. His coal-black hair is blow-dried. With his white tennis shorts and red polo shirt, he is the gay neighbor most families never knew they had. Articulate with a deep baritone, his accent places his childhood somewhere in New England.

The Expo is Doug's first entrance into the positive community as an HIV-positive individual. It is a coming-out party of sorts. Up until today, the only people who knew about his status were his doctor, his business partner, a good friend who is also positive, and his HIV-negative boyfriend.

Like Tim in Chapter 2, who opened up to his positive NA group, by arriving at a place created for and by HIV-positive individuals, Doug is starting the process of acceptance and healing. At the same time, his relationship with his new boyfriend, Jake, is also just beginning: "We had only been dating for six weeks before I tested HIV positive, and it was, I think, a bigger deal for me than for him." Doug describes what happened when he disclosed his status to Jake: "He was very supportive the night that I told him. I insisted that we spend a week apart after that, without any communication, so that he could think it all through on his own, weigh the pros and cons, and all that." When the week was over, Jake still wanted to continue with their relationship.

Doug, on the other hand, is still holding back: "I'm still coming to terms with all of the ramifications of being HIV-positive. I am in a redefining position right now, a rediscovery position, and I can't, haven't come to any conclusions yet. I can't put words to how I have changed or how I am changing." He also doesn't know if Jake will still be a part of his life when he is finished changing. Because Doug is not sure of what he wants yet, he has pulled back just in case he says or does something irretrievable.

Doug wants some time to work things out. Because he has just been diagnosed, he realizes that he is in the process of changing. He wants the time and space to figure out how he will live the rest of his life—romantically, emotionally, spiritually, and careerwise. Deciding whether or not he wants Jake to be there with him in the long run is part of that decision. Doug wonders if this love will be his last. If so, does he want to have his last love be with someone whom he has to hold back sexually for, given that Jake is negative? It also made him assess what he valued and didn't value in his partner and their relationship. "Once I became aware that I was positive," he says, "it just made me think, 'If my lifespan is going to be shortened, is this the person I *definitely* want to spend the rest of it with?' You know, it makes all those little questions that you normally ask about a relationship—at least, for me—it's made them even more important."

Doug has entered a transformative period, and in a different sense so has Jake. All the hypothetical questions that lurk in the background of gay men's lives—"How would I handle my relationships with HIV-negative men if I were diagnosed HIV-positive?"; "What if I remained negative and suddenly found out that a partner I'd made a commitment to was positive?"—have suddenly leaped into the foreground. In answering these questions, Doug and Jake have a chance to turn the crisis before them into an opportunity for growth—of themselves and also their relationship. But it will take time, soul-searching thought, and candid communication.

Should your last love be someone you have to hold back sexually for?

This chapter looks at the answers that different men have arrived at. Because positive–negative relationships, whether they're one-night stands or long-term commitments, are a fact of life for virtually all of us, we've addressed this configuration first, and much of what we discuss in this chapter applies to everyone. No matter what your serostatus or who your partners are, it is important to look at not only how to navigate safer sex but also how to understand your neighbors and lovers who are on the other side of the HIV fence.

Anxiety, HIV, and Sex: The New Three-Way

Some couples have reported that being in a relationship where at least one of the partners is positive is easier because HIV becomes a known element. The presumption (which it often can be) of negative status does not exist. In other words, many negative partners feel that if they were not in a relationship and were out in the dating world, they would be more likely to let down their guard, meet people who do not disclose or do not know their status, have more partners, have more sex, and hence be at greater risk for seroconversion.

On the other hand, some describe the lovemaking between a couple of mixed serostatus as a *menage à trois* because there never is a time when HIV is not present in the bedroom. The anxiety this produces can serve the couple well in maintaining the negative status of one partner and keeping the positive partner safer from opportunistic disease, but it can certainly create other challenges in the couple's relationship.

Where Did the Passion Go?

A common complaint about long-term relationships is the reduction in sexual activity—a shift from not being able to keep your hands off each other to lowered interest in lovemaking as the relationship proceeds. Whether your relationship is short- or long-term, lower testosterone levels, depression, and overall disease progression can definitely put a damper on your sex life when one of you is diagnosed HIV positive. If this change disturbs you, talk to your physician, who should be sensitive to how changes in the body affect not only the patient but his partner as well.

But before you attribute any change in your sex life to your new position as a mixed-status couple, try to ascertain whether this change had been coming already as a consequence of both longevity and comfortable familiarity you have with your partner. This natural sequence in most couples lives is a shift from an initial period of intense sexual activity to having a more companionate type of relationship. If you're a long-term couple, you may already have begun expressing your intimacy in different ways that do not involve sex, such as kissing and holding one another. Or maybe there was a disparity in your individual sex drives, as there is between Doug and Jake.

> **Before you attribute any change in your sex life to your new position as a mixed-status couple, try to ascertain whether this change had been coming already as a consequence of both longevity and comfortable familiarity you have with your partner.**

Because Doug is asymptomatic, the couple's issues surrounding sex are nonmedical. When diagnosed, Doug, like many others, felt a decrease in his libido, mostly because he is scared of transmitting the disease to his partner, a man for whom he cares deeply (see the box). The two instead have begun to explore other kinds of intimacy and sensuality. Their other stumbling block is a difference in sexual taste. Doug has a much wider palette than Jake. "I like a lot of sex. I'm just a very sensual, sexual person," he says in his patrician Boston accent. He acknowledges the contradictions in his dilemma. The positive diagnosis makes him feel like a non-

> An excellent website that looks at ways in which HIV-positive men take an active approach to keeping their partners negative is located at *www.HIVStopswithme.org.*

sexual person, and yet he assumes that at some point he will again feel comfortable being sexually active. For now, they cuddle and give each other massages. But, as Doug admits a little guiltily, "It's still very Donna Reed."

Doug realizes and appreciates Jake's patience. Doug has stepped back emotionally, romantically, and sexually, and he knows this is hard on Jake. He keeps thinking to himself, "Just another couple of weeks and I'll have this figured out." Whether he will may depend on several factors including not only what he envisions in what he wants in a partner but also whether he is ready for a re-

If passion has waned, is HIV really to blame?

lationship. Whatever decision he comes to as an individual, he will benefit from the knowledge that he had the experience of being in a relationship where he was accepted for who he is, recognizing that HIV is only one part of the equation.

Even when the HIV-positive partner has symptoms of the disease, some couples see a return to sex as treatment regimens such as the testosterone gel rekindle a diminishing sex drive and restore lean muscle mass and physical appearance. Androgenic steroidal agents have their downside, however, and should be used only after carefully weighing their potential systemic effect on the psyche and the rest of the body. Sure, they can enhance muscular growth and stimulate the sex drive, but these effects sometimes leave men feeling deceptively invincible. Some of the agents are toxic to the liver, which is a major site of metabolism for many of the antiretroviral drugs. In other words, they may make you feel like a new man while they are actually harming your medication's power to stave off HIV-related illness.

Dual Risks, Dual Responsibilities

Doug describes how Jake's "behavior almost indicated that I had never told him. I mean he was doing things that were flirting with risk"—he lowers his voice to a whisper—"you know, sexually."

When Doug confronted his boyfriend about this, Jake responded, "Well, I've been thinking about it, and sometimes I think it would be better if I just went ahead and became positive too, and that way we wouldn't have this issue anymore."

Doug thinks, "That's right, *we* wouldn't have this issue, but *you* would have a whole new one, and it would come with an earlier expiration date than you had probably planned." Doug understands wanting the certainty that being positive brings, so that every time you become intimate it is not yet another crapshoot, always questioning: Will the condom break this time? Will I stay negative one more day? With these queries comes the underlying question: Will I have to watch this love die while I stay healthy?

While Jake's logic is ill advised, many negatives who date positives can relate to the sentiment of wanting to put their partners at ease. They do not want the positive person to have to worry so much about the transmission. There are better things to worry about, such as staying healthy.

Doug, however, wants no part in spreading the disease to one more person, especially to a person he cares for. At any rate, Jake's attitude concerns Doug. He is not sure that he wants to continue a relationship with someone willing to put himself at risk. That attitude has added to the dampening of Doug's sexual desire.

Doug realizes that not only must he work on full acceptance of his disease but he must also share these skills with his partner(s). Whether Doug and Jake remain together, using the proper precautions—from the moment of disclosure onward—requires both parties to be equally vigilant about protection.

Safer Sex: Intimacy Insurance

"Put your legs up, over your shoulders. That's it," Brian breathlessly instructs Justin as they lie naked in bed. Justin stops him. "Wait. In school we had this lecture about safe sex." Brian replies confidently, "And now we're going to have a demonstration." Brian reaches for a condom, tears it open with his mouth, and gives it to Justin. "Put it on me. Go on. Slip it on."

—Showtime's *Queer as Folk* premier episode,
December 2000

No sex is completely safe in the presence of HIV, which is why protective measures are referred to collectively as "saf*er* sex," no longer as "safe sex." The following pages explain how positive–negative couples can engage in safer sex today. Understanding this early on is vital, especially if you have been socialized like many men to engage in sex early in a relationship.

Following the guidelines in this section will help you minimize sexual risk (see the accompanying box). *Safer sex precautions are necessary even when all evidence indicates that both you and your partner(s) are completely healthy.* This is why everyone should read this section, not just HIV-negatives who have positive partners, full time or occasionally, or HIV-positives with negative partners.

Safer Sex: Guidelines

TWO-WAY STREET

While you may be determined to keep your lovers healthy, your partners need to be equally diligent in not passing anything to you. Also, just because he says he is HIV negative, the result is only as good as the last time he got tested. Independent of your HIV status, if you are sexually active, it is important to get regular checkups for sexually transmitted infections. Be sure to ask your health care provider to perform these tests, as this is not part of a traditional physical.

> **When was the last time your partner was tested? The safety of being negative expires on the date of the most recent test.**

USE CONDOMS

The single most effective thing you can do to stay healthy while being sexually active is to use latex condoms for intercourse (whether vaginal, if you are bisexual, or anal). When you put on a condom, pinch its tip as you unroll it (all the way down) to prevent an air bubble from forming in the reservoir tip. For intercourse, you should then put some water-based lubricant on the outside of the condom for comfort, mutual pleasure, and to keep the condom from tearing during sex. It's very important to hold on to the base of the condom as you withdraw (after becoming soft) so it doesn't slip off. For those with latex allergies, polyurethane condoms are available. Those made of lambskin are too porous to prevent HIV.

ORAL SEX

While opinions may differ on the level of risk from oral sex, there is no doubt that precautions are warranted. One approach is flavored and nonlubricated condoms. Evidence suggests that the risk of transmitting HIV is considered much lower for unprotected oral sex than for unprotected anal intercourse. The risk is lowest for the recipient, and for the person performing oral sex the risk of transmission is lower if his mouth and gums are healthy and if his partner doesn't ejaculate in his mouth. Be careful in this last instance, for preejaculation is common. Some sex educators recommend not flossing or brushing your teeth an hour before you perform oral sex (you can use antibacterial mouthwash if you're concerned about bad breath), and others recommend quickly looking over the genitals of your partner for signs of contagious sexually transmitted diseases (STDs). (Again, these precautions were considered valid as of the time of publication but may change in the future.)

Some sex educators also suggest that if while performing unprotected fellatio your partner does ejaculate in your mouth, it's better to immediately spit out the semen than to either wait or swallow it, and it may help (especially for bacterial STDs) to promptly go use an antibacterial or peroxide mouthwash.

VACCINATIONS

There are two STDs for which permanent vaccines are available: hepatitis B and hepatitis A. Hepatitis B can be spread easily through intercourse and (less easily) through oral sex or rimming (anal–oral contact). Hepatitis A is easily spread through rimming. Getting the hepatitis B vaccination would be an excellent idea if you don't always use barriers for these activities. Hepatitis A is sometimes age dependent and should be discussed with your physician; if the doctor approves, you can get both vaccinations at the same time. A vaccine to prevent HIV currently is being developed, and options may exist in your area to participate in clinical trials. (No HIV vaccine has as yet been proved effective, however.)

DISCLOSURE

Disclosure may prevent your partner from contracting the disease if you're the one who is currently positive, but it affords a number of other protections for you. Though we ranked the safer-sex behaviors in the box on the facing page, please note that there is limited scientific information available to solidly rank the risk of behaviors.

High risk[1]

- *Receptive anal intercourse without a condom.* This means having a man put his penis in your anus without using a condom (rubber). This is even riskier if he ejaculates (cums).

- *Insertive anal intercourse without a condom.* This means putting your penis in someone's anus without a condom.

- *Sharing uncovered sex toys (dildos, anal beads, etc.).* This means putting the same sex toy in your own and your partner's anus.

NOTE: *Fisting (insertion of the hand or fist into the anus)* can increase the risk of HIV transmission when combined with any of the activities listed above.

- *Rimming (oral–anal contact)* substantially increases the risk of transmission of diseases caused by other organisms such as Giardia and hepatitis virus A.

Some risk

- *Oral sex with a man without a condom.* This means giving (higher risk) or getting a blow job without using a condom. This is especially risky if the man ejaculates.

- *Receptive anal intercourse with a condom.* This means having someone put his penis in your anus while using a condom.

- *Insertive anal intercourse with a condom.* This means putting your penis in someone's anus while using a condom.

- *Finger or hand stimulation of your partner's genitals if you have cuts on your hands.*

Little risk

- *Oral sex with men with a condom.* This means giving or getting a blow job while wearing a condom (rubber).

- *Deep (French) kissing.* While saliva does not transmit HIV, the presence of blood due to bleeding gums or cuts may increase the risk of transmission.

No risk

- *Erotic massage, hugging, mutual masturbation (without cuts on the hands), body-to-body rubbing, fantasy.*

Although it can be hard, you have a moral and ethical obligation to inform all sex and needle-sharing partners of your HIV infection. It may also be in your best interest to inform them to avoid future legal problems, depending on where you live (see Appendix A for more information as to legal issues).

You may know about these practices and be an ardent practitioner of them but find yourself getting trapped in a cycle of frequent, short-term sexual partners that is now leaving you feeling emotionally ungratified. The significant risk in having sex early on is greatest if you are not disclosing your status—a topic to which we have devoted all of Chapter 1.

With nondisclosure comes the added risk of losing your partner completely. Backtracking is difficult to do when it comes to someone believing in you. Sharing and trust are especially vital for us if we want to have a positive (in all its meanings) and enduring relationship. *Enduring* is a word that I challenge you to refamiliarize yourself with, as I challenge myself, as men with HIV live longer lives and hence longer love lives.

PEP Talk: Postexposure Prophylaxis—Is It the New "Morning-After" Treatment?

When you're involved in a positive–negative relationship, even safer sex is risky. A tear in whatever latex you might be using can lead to accidental exposure to the virus. Because of new preemptive therapies, however, exposure may not invariably result in infection.

Much discussion has arisen about a misnamed morning-after treatment, or more accurately *postexposure prophylaxis* (PEP; see the box), which has been available for a while to some health care workers exposed to HIV-infected blood in the line of duty (through needle pricks and the like). The treatment isn't necessarily performed the morning after someone is exposed, but it is provided before the health

National PEP Hotline, 1-888-HIV-4911, is a resource for clinicians who need treatment information for their patients. The general public may call the Centers for Disease Control and Prevention (CDC) National AIDS Hotline at 1-800-342-2437 for providers in their area who offer counseling and treatment for those who may have been recently exposed. (En Español: 1-800-344-7432.)

care workers test positive, in the hope of preventing exposure to the disease from automatically becoming an infection by using all of the new protease inhibitors as quickly as possible after first exposure. If the treatment becomes commonplace for non-health-care workers as well, it could ease the anxiety involved in negative–positive sexual relations by giving serodiscordant couples hope that tears in latex will not necessarily cause infection.

WILL PEP WORK, AND SHOULD IT BE USED MORE WIDELY?

The theory is that protease inhibitors prevent the virus from entering the host cell, and because the virus cannot survive very long on its own without cells to hide out in, the hope is to prevent the exposure from becoming an infection. So it is assumed that protease inhibitors will stop the AIDS viruses from reproducing and therefore stop them from taking root in the blood and other systems in the body. One belief is that with this early treatment, exposure does not necessitate infection.

The morning-after treatment directed at AIDS has, of course, started the same kind of controversy that arose when the "morning-after pill" was developed for use immediately after intercourse to prevent pregnancy by inducing abortion. If you make it widely available, critics claim, irresponsible people will rely on it instead of using safer-sex practices or clean needles. Doctors and public health officials also argue that wide distribution of the drugs could encourage the mutation of a drug-resistant strain within the bodies of people who do not take the drugs as directed—at the right times, eating or not eating when they are supposed to. (The mechanism is the same as for antibiotics taken for a sinus infection or strep throat. If you stop taking the medicine before you finish it because you are feeling better, you leave some of the bacteria in your system, and they will come back full force once the antibiotic is absent, sometimes stronger than before. The concern regarding PEP is that, as has happened with multi-drug-resistant tuberculosis, an HIV strain will develop that does not respond to treatment.) In addition, physicians are cautious about prescribing them to people who do not react well to the drug therapies. Finally, they offer the notion that it is unclear whether or not this treatment will work the same for sexual transmission as it does for a needle transmission.

On the other side of the debate are many AIDS activists, as well

Who should receive postexposure prophylaxis— and who should have the power to decide?

as Ralph Nader's Public Citizen group, who are calling for the preemptive therapy to be available to the public to stop the spread of AIDS. If this treatment can stop exposure from becoming an infection, the prodistribution folks' thinking is that we can at least slow down the spread of the virus a bit as well as prevent some individuals from getting the disease; even if the therapy just slows down the process of the disease within these individuals, it will give them a chance to survive until a cure is found.

What is really going on in the minds of the "experts," say the AIDS activists, is moral judgment. Doctors and nurses are the "we" in their arguments: good people trying to help the masses. The "them"—the others to whom the treatment is not available—are irresponsible, bad people who spread the AIDS virus and who cannot be trusted to take the medicine as they should.

In response to the perceived weakness in the argument against providing PEP to the general public, a few private physicians are making it available. The San Francisco Health Department has implemented a public program in that city making this treatment available to the general public. Visit your local urgent care center or AIDS Service Organization to see if they provide this service, or if you can get an immediate appointment with your doctor contact him or her. The risk in this scenario is that your primary care physician may not be knowledgeable about this option and won't know how to proceed. Anticipating that scenario, I have included a National PEP Hotline number that is geared to clinicians in the box on page 68—it may help to provide your physician that number.

A PREEMPTIVE STRIKE IN THE BATTLE AGAINST HIV

In Washington, DC, Dr. I. M. Bruni,[2] an infectious disease specialist, is working to make this morning-after treatment, or (as he prefers to call it) *preemptive therapy,* available to the public. Dr. Bruni formed his philosophy about preemptive therapy several years ago, when a patient called from a business trip in Iowa. This patient described his symptoms over the phone: "I'm sick. I've got a sore throat, and I've got a rash. I'm having fevers, and my lymph nodes are swollen"—the symptoms of acute AIDS. These are also the symptoms of several other diseases. A doctor in Iowa had diagnosed this man's symptoms as the chicken pox. Having already had chicken pox as a child (he could remember the year and date and offered to call his mother to confirm them), the patient suspected it was something else. Dr. Bruni suspected it was acute HIV infection and urged the patient to come in for treatment.

When the CDC came out with guidelines for setting up preemptive therapy for medical workers, Dr. Bruni started to advertise in the local gay paper, the *Washington Blade*. The ads, for the most part, reflected the public service ads: "Get tested, Get treated." But they also included "Think you've been exposed recently?"

Dr. Bruni does not have much patience for doctors and other experts who give "excuses" for not prescribing preemptive therapy to those who are exposed to the disease through sexual encounters or through drug use. Where others see the morning-after treatment as a possible public health risk (by encouraging the development of a drug-resistant strain), Dr. Bruni thinks about his responsibility to his individual patients. His response to the argument that a person who is irresponsible enough to consistently engage in risky behaviors is unlikely to follow the proper treatment regimen and is therefore at greater risk for developing drug-resistant strains is that if you stop the spread of the disease in just one person's bloodstream, you will stop the possibility of it being passed on to another person. In other words, by preventing infection in one person, you prevent the exposure and infection to countless others, especially if that one person continuously engages in risky behavior.

Important in Dr. Bruni's medical practice and medical philosophy is open and nonjudgmental dialogue between the patient and the doctor. This dialogue gives the doctor more of an idea of how to treat his patients, but it also gives the patients a place to get new information. Dr. Bruni does not initially tell his patients how to have safe sex, but he does answer any questions they might have about safe sex. This way he becomes a source of information instead of someone who dispenses pills and speeches. He does not want to give the "you should have known better" speech, because, as he says, "that . . . doesn't do anything except close down the communication." The communication is very important, he says, especially if you are seeing someone for the first time or if that patient has never spoken to anyone about HIV or even the possibility of HIV.

Have Current Treatments Created a New Sexual Overconfidence?

The new treatments are extending our lives for years beyond what those diagnosed HIV positive could once hope for. But they are also fostering a new sexual confidence that has the potential to undo much of the good done by today's protease inhibitors. Many men have come to believe that if a person is on the protease inhibitors and his viral load is undetectable in his bloodstream, then the virus, by the same logic, must be undetectable in his semen and therefore he is no longer contagious (see the box). Dr. Troy P. Suarez, director of scientific services at MediSolutions in New York City, leading a team of researchers, conducted a survey of 472 HIV-negative men attending a gay pride festival to determine if perceived risk changes depending on that partner's disclosed HIV status, antiretroviral status, and viral load. Of the different possible scenarios, sex with an HIV-positive man not taking medication was viewed as posing the greatest risk. Sex with an HIV-positive partner who was taking medication and had an undetectable viral load *was not consistently viewed as riskier* than sex with an HIV-negative partner or a man of unknown HIV status. The findings suggest that gay and bisexual men may be more prone to have unprotected sex with someone on medication than with those who are not.[4]

In reviewing this study the most striking component was the concept of "perception of risk" and how we as

> In a 1999 issue of *The Hopkins HIV Report*, Richard J. Pomerantz, MD, director of the Center for Human Virology, noted that he could "find no correlation between the amount of HIV in an individual's blood and the quantity found in sperm."[3]

positive men hear the word *undetectable*. Along with the HIV-negative men in the Suarez study, many positive men have come to view their lab results as the excuse they have been waiting for not to use condoms or practice safer sex any longer. When our doctors gave us our pills, which led to an undetectable viral load, it did not mean that we now could clear off the space on our medicine cabinet formerly occupied by our condoms. Serodiscordant couples who are returning to sex without condoms are taking a life-threatening chance. *Let there be no doubt about it: any amount of the virus, whether detectable in the bloodstream or not, is assumed to be sufficient to infect a sexual partner.*[5]

Only time will tell, however, what long-term ramifications the assumption will have that men who are on medication are safer sexual partners. Are we forming a new sexual hierarchy that includes subcategories for those with access to new treatments? Are we beginning to blur the clear division between the positives and the negatives? Will those seeking partners now give preference to those with undetectable viral loads over those who may be further along in their disease progression?

Differences and Similarities: HIV as a Factor in the Shaping of a Relationship

In my work with couples, I've found that most got together either unaware of their serostatus or knowing, from previous tests, that they were both negative. When that shared status changed for one of them, the survival of the relationship was often threatened. The problems that ensue when both partners have known their status all along and the HIV-positive individual hasn't revealed his status right away are obvious: whatever trust had grown between them may now be dashed. But other times it's illness, routine follow-up, or retesting that identifies one partner as positive. As I've said, motivations for waiting to be tested can be complicated, possibly having to do with the fear of discovering the virus without having the backup of a supportive partner. Increasingly, couples are agreeing that both will get tested earlier than was once common, often less than six months into the relationship—perhaps as a rite of passage to a next level of intimacy, knowledge, and trust.

However the discovery of serodiscordance comes about, it invariably creates a crisis within the couple. Whether it will translate into the couple's drawing closer together or breaking up is difficult to forecast, though that can often be predicted by their level of open communication and mutual trust prior to the crisis.

A more fundamental problem may be that serodiscordance exaggerates the inherent differences that already exist between any two partners. The medical crisis demands our attention right now and may push the underlying emotional issues into the background: How will we deal with the fact that we are no longer as similar as we once thought? Will this change the balance of power? Will it shift roles in ways that we can adapt to? While we're understandably worrying about the fate of the positive partner and the risk for the currently negative partner, who's worrying about the stability of the relationship?

Who's minding the relationship while you're both worrying about physical health and risk?

In coupling with anyone else we are entering a personal and shared intimacy with an inherently different person. When looking at potential partners we examine how different that person is from us and from those around us, and in what ways he is similar and can be integrated into our daily lives and shared social interactions. Partners who have never been involved with someone of different serostatus before may have more trouble adjusting to this momentous shift in what has been shared between them so far. Partners who started out assuming (accurately or not) that they were both negative may have been basking in the coupled bliss of feeling as if they've found their soul mate, that one person who was a perfect fit—usually because of perceived similarities more than differences. Many may not even be aware of the other person being different or "other" until they know their serostatus through disclosure. At that point, though, this person has already begun to be integrated into their lives: they are either head over heels in love or starting to fall in love.

Now that a huge difference has been unveiled, will "love conquer all"? If all factors are equal, or more precisely ideal, will the presence or absence of HIV in one's bloodstream (and other bodily fluids) create an insurmountable challenge or something a couple can indeed face together? The term *discordant couple*, while referring to serostatus, implies that this difference will create discord and conflict and seems to act as a predictor of an unhappy, if not doomed, relationship. Yet many couples do get closer when the crisis befalls them, and we now know that this cohesion is often instrumental in the sta-

Will the crisis of seroconversion pull you apart or draw you together?

bilization of the positive partner. Both partners need to call on their emotional resources to assist themselves and each other in alleviating new fears, anxieties, and the potential specters of illness and death.

Taking Control of the Time Warp

As Doug explained earlier, the seroconversion of one member of a couple can force both to confront their mortality; the illness and death that were once so distant are now frighteningly close. This can plunge the couple into a time warp that often compromises their ability to weather the crisis together. How a couple navigates, negotiates, and understands time is critical to the rhythm of the relationship. Yet strategies that are integral to successful relationships such as the setting of long-term goals may suddenly seem difficult, if not pointless.

Are you rushing toward intimacy because time suddenly seems so short?

Have you come to a complete standstill because you no longer see the point in moving toward the future?

The newly serodiscordant couple may suffer from time distortions that speed things up, at least for the HIV-positive partner ("I have so little time that I want to do as much as possible") or slow them to a halt ("I'm just waiting to die"). A heightened sense of living for today may bring a positive new vigor to the couple's lives, or it may thrust them into a fast lane from which it can be hard to escape. The couple that wants to experience all the intimacy they can right now might feel a sense of urgency to enter into and move through the phases of coupling more quickly than the relationship can withstand. This phenomenon is also discussed in Chapter 4 as a relationship dynamic that occurs often with positive–positive couples.

Fortunately, some couples become aware that their intimacy is accelerating too quickly, and either individually or as a couple they take steps to moderate this and pursue a slower pace. Doug's hesitance to pursue intimacy with Jake and his alarm at Jake's apparent willingness to sacrifice his own health to be with Doug without anxiety are examples of the way some individuals step back during this crisis. Whether Doug and Jake's relationship survives the crisis may depend on whether they can recognize their time discordance and get back into synch with each other. If you feel that you and your partner are out of rhythm with each other after one of you is diagnosed with HIV, it's important to look at the disparity and discuss it with reassurance and confidence that the relationship will move forward.

Sometimes "speediness" isn't aimed at the relationship but at one person's efforts to deal with the pressing sense of mortality. Some people increase their alcohol intake or drug abuse upon being diagnosed with HIV, justifying it as a way to handle the fear or actual experience of diminished health. If you or your partner is engaging in such destructive behavior, look seriously at whether this is something that you or your partner can resolve. Also consider getting professional help and ongoing support to address the underlying and ongoing issues that triggered this. Also I encourage you to reread Chapter 2, where we examine this very question and offer strategies to aid you with this.

For the terminally ill, a pain avoidance approach does have elements of logic to it. However, ways in which people go about it are different. As a strong believer in pain management in advanced stages of illness (as best seen in hospice care or by compassionate health care providers), I understand the need to "escape." Substance abuse occurs when these pain-avoiding behaviors are unduly preemptive—to put it more plainly, this is like taking an aspirin before the headache occurs.

Time can be distorted in the other direction as well. A lethargic and depressed response is usually expressed in withdrawal from intimacy and refusal to pursue life with enthusiasm and gusto. Obviously this transformation can be painful to witness. If you are the HIV-negative partner of a man who has plunged into severe depression and has suddenly lost all of his fighting spirit, you may respond with forced cheerfulness, which may deplete you emotionally and carries the risk of creating an artificial wedge between the two of you.

What's your response to a positive partner's depression and lethargy—forced cheerfulness, aggression, escape through abuse of drugs or alcohol?

Some men, in extreme cases, resort to violence, literally trying to shake their partner out of this depression. While often driven by desperation and often fear, physical violence or emotional abuse is an unacceptable response. If an unexpected or uncharacteristic burst of violence occurs, support and couples counseling may be an appropriate and targeted response. The goal and intervention would be to address the underlying stressors that prompted this emotional eruption at it earliest stages. However, if abuse is an on-going dynamic within your relationship and you have fears either now for your own safety or that you may not control your anger, a trial seperation may be in order. The goal once again is to mediate the stressors that created this situation or develop a personal safety plan leading to a recognition that while the relationship is not sal-vageable, your personal dignity and safety are.

If your partner has allowed his life to come to a standstill now that HIV has intruded, you may find it helpful to gain an under-standing of the disease process and how other couples synchronize their lives in response to it. In later chapters we will look at the ways couples navigate their relationship when illness is more pro-nounced. We will also look at issues of caregiving and the feelings of grief and loss that can occur even prior to death of a partner.

Role Confusion and Power Struggles

The supreme happiness of life is conviction that we are
loved–loved for ourselves, or in spite of ourselves.
                                        —Victor Hugo, *Les Misérables*

Relationships are often evaluated from a power-based perspective, perhaps because in the traditional heterosexual relationship the man had more power due to physical strength, earning potential, and societal values. Within couples of mixed serostatus, often there are feelings of powerlessness for the negative partner as well as the one who is directly facing ill health and a life-threatening illness. Discord may enter into the relationship in response to medical treatment decisions, noncompliance with treatment, and other pragmatic matters. But for most serodiscordant couples the role confusions and power struggles have to do more generally with issues of caretaking, dependence, the risk of infecting the negative partner, and guilt. These issues are complicated to unravel, and what makes them more difficult is that they usually shift and change over time.

Stephen, a thirty-two-year-old HIV-negative former patient of mine, stated about his lover, "Joe is kind of lackadaisical about taking his pills on time. The protease inhibitor is

Can the two of you agree on medical decisions and compliance with treatment, or is the cure starting to cause more conflict than the disease?

one [he needs to be] very strict about when to take it, when he eats, etc. His carefree attitude was one thing that attracted me to him when we were younger—I was such a worrywart back then and still am. I get angry because I want him in my life and I don't want to end up being his caretaker prematurely because he won't do what he is supposed to do. He is very good at going to his acupuncture and massage appointments, but the follow-through on these meds, that's a different story."

Views on medicine and the level and type of investment that a person who is negative puts into his partner's care may put unique strains on a couple. This conflict doesn't exist for single people, who can make these decisions independently. These issues will need to be discussed if you decide to make your romantic partner the person responsible for health care decisions (see Appendix A) when you are unable to make your own. Also, many people who are positive fear becoming a burden on their partners or having them watch as their illness progresses. They fear not being able to be full and equal partners in the relationship.

Power roles can also become revised as the one who is positive begins to make more requests of the one who is negative. This may occur even prior to the decline in health status. These requests may not even be clearly voiced, but the negative partner may acquiesce more readily when they are and inadvertently create an unhealthy environment in an attempt to avoid conflict and stress. Arguments that may have occurred in the past get squelched, and acquiescence becomes more regular, creating an artificial harmony that is difficult to maintain in the long run. Which is when those who are positive *really need you to be there*—in the long run. Hence the ability to have candid nonattacking discussions is a critical skill for any couple, independent of serostatus.

The HIV-positive partner who fears that his partner won't be there for him or who fears that caretaking may be an unwanted burden may find himself wanting to end the relationship. Choices in responding to both crisis and conflict invariably break down to a "fight-or-flight" response. A flight response may often be triggered by concern for the partner or attempt to control and anticipate a possible outcome. One feared outcome is that your partner will not be there at the moment when you need him most. Leaving the relationship acts as a preemptive strike. Doug exemplifies the internal struggle between fight and flight responses when he struggles with whether to stay in his new supportive relationship with Jake or to back away and pull the plug on the relationship before it ends of its own accord.

Does the idea of leaving your HIV-negative partner so that you won't become a burden to him sound like a noble idea? Is it beginning to seem like a viable plan?

This desire to flee, whether for "noble" purposes or from fear, requires the couple to anticipate/plan how they will progress through the disease together and what will be the ways to do this with as much grace and forethought as possible. While it is important to recognize the instinct to flee, if the relationship is basically sound, a measured practical response may be what is really needed. Also, consulting an objective third party such as a therapist or gay-sensitive minister may be warranted.

Caretaker or Codependent?

Another term for the serodiscordant couple is the *magnetic couple.* While this term is obviously meant to refer to the positive and negative status of the two, it implies an irresistible attraction to someone of a different HIV status. Some men actually may choose a positive partner intentionally, based on their self-image as caretakers or as people who are unable to have a long-term relationship. If one of your core beliefs is that relationships don't last (perhaps stemming from your being the child of divorced parents) or if you buy into the society's message that gay men are unable to form and maintain relationships, would you unconsciously choose a partner who expects a shorter lifespan, hence expecting some sort a self-fulfilling prophecy? This type of thinking needs to be challenged not only in how it is affecting your relationship but with the added understanding that new treatments mean longer and healthier lives. A relationship that relies unduly on HIV as a type of emotional glue to maintain the relationship (in this new reality) may be destined for trouble. Therefore, if your relationships in the past have lasted only so long, either you may have developed a resilient nature that focuses on the ability to heal and begin once more or you have habitually not invested in the relationships with sufficient depth and time, prompting them to end prematurely. Relationships, like all living things, have a natural rhythm and life to them. HIV often robs us of that. In the end, remember you are both the guardian and warden of your own heart and must determine not only whom to let in but also when it is time to let go.

You may be a natural caretaker with a compassionate outlook toward others if you come from a culture or individual background in which you have experienced oppression and stigma. As a child you may have come from a nurturing and affirming family where you were exposed to ways of showing and receiving care without resentment. The capacity to become involved with a positive partner may present a host of opportunities and challenges. Either you could end up being an effective caretaker when the time comes (the healthier scenario) or you could end up being codependent. The ability to be a caring partner, able to care for yourself along with your positive partner, will be markedly different from an unhealthy codependency. This dynamic is something I explore more fully later in Chapter 6, when we consider what is a healthy relationship and how we as men are able to not only give but receive nurturance when our (or our partner's) physical health is challenged.

> **Have your relationships been short lived in the past? If so, are you naturally resilient, able to start over with optimism, or are you simply investing too little time and depth to make them grow?**

On the other hand, if either of you is overwhelmed by the positive partner's and the couple's needs or if you are afraid to ask for help and support, you run the risk of ending up in a relationship of excessive dependency, which may lead to resentment and guilt. One possible response to this for many gay men has been to create broad-based friendship networks that duplicate many of the functions of the traditional family. Feeling free and willing to call on friends and receive nurturance as a couple is integral to preventing burnout (an idea that is discussed further in Chapter 6). The couple creates a built-in network that is available as a resource for them from dating, to what were once the inevitable specters of disability and death, to the real possibility of seeing themselves grow into old married men together.

FOUR

AN INDIAN SUMMER ROMANCE
Positives with Positives

Seroharmonious—that was the word my former partner Jerry and I used to describe our relationship. Relationships are ideally ones in which harmony is more prevalent than conflict and discord. *Seroharmonious* roughly translates as "same blood" and is the antonym of *serodiscordant* ("different blood"). Seroharmonious described our relationship in that the blood that flowed through both our hearts was HIV positive.

Reflecting on my relationship in the context of the work I have done with other "harmonious" couples, it seems as if our relationship had a quality different from the much-hyped spring fever romances. Ours had a spirit more consistent with Indian summer—a time of year that is very much aware of the upcoming winter. With an intensity of trees ablaze in fiery reds and provocative golds, it had a passion that a summer romance cannot know. Playing in leaves, raking yards, and wearing big wool sweaters, the need and expectations to get closer, to hold tightly, to stay warm—this is autumn.

Similarity Breeds Empathy

If the basic premise of homosexuality is attraction to our own, is the phenomenon of choosing positive partners a variation on or a continuation of this theme? Commonality of life experience has always been one of the great human connections. So when HIV-positive people say, "I want someone with whom I have something in common," what is shared often incorporates some aspect of HIV.

Illness as a life experience can bring people together in many ways. In a 1986 survey of 150 people with spinal injury, multiple sclerosis, or stroke, two-thirds of the respondents felt that their disability had given them opportunities to form new friendships with others like them, "through consumer organizations and self-help groups, increased time for and increased interest in friendships as compared with predisability relationships."[1] The authors of the book *Dynamics of Relationships* said "the common knowledge of the illness experience provides a rather special kind of bond."[2] But it isn't just common experience—which fosters empathy and intimacy—that throws HIV positives together. Positives choose to couple with each other for other reasons as well, some of which stem from fear: fear of discrimination for having HIV, which can cause isolation, and the fear of infecting negative people.

In other words, having HIV in common can go a long way. It can be self-serving in that the commonality makes partners more knowledgeable about their own illness and better able to act as advocates for their own health care. It can simply act as a convenience at times when one doesn't feel like going to the drugstore and can borrow a partner's AZT (azidothymidine) or protease inhibitors.

As you read on, however, you'll discover that coupling with someone just because he is positive can also spell trouble in a relationship. It can place a special burden on the relationship when both people are ill or when one partner is more ill than the other. The amount of stress the couple experiences may create an unexpected distance between them as the illness causes shifts in roles, power, and expectations. These shifts may not have been anticipated adequately when the two originally coupled, though both were aware of their HIV-positive status.

Coupling and Connecting as a Health Benefit

Numerous studies have pointed to the concrete health benefits of being in a coupled relationship—something that is especially important for someone who is ill. The work of Kiecolt-Glaser et al. (1985) suggests that supportive relationships may have an impact on overall immune functioning: "The implication is that the presence or absence of supportive relationships may alter immune function in a manner that may place individuals at lower risk for illness onset or illness progression."[3]

For straight couples who have been together for a lifetime or who have been very closely enmeshed, when the husband or the wife dies, the remaining spouse runs a higher risk of dying soon afterward, due to depression and loss of the will to live, which can bring on illness. Consider also a male couple, both HIV-positive, who coupled soon before one succumbed to AIDS. The survivor, who before his lover's death staunchly fought the disease mentally, then realized and accepted the possibility of his own death and died six months later.

Men with supportive relationships may lower their risk of illness progression.

Isolation—not having a sense of connection to a family, community or individual—can contribute to depression (see the box), a variety of stressors, and other illnesses. In fact, numerous studies have shown that those with chronic illnesses, including AIDS, isolate themselves much more than do those without chronic illnesses. The onset of disability often results in a decrease in social interaction—less contact with friends, especially those who may have been part of your health support network. Fatigue often occurs for one's support system, as it does for the person who is ill. Initially, after being diagnosed, one may receive a lot of support, but that often decreases as the illness progresses. A good example is when someone is hospitalized for the first time, compared to the fifth hospitalization: the first time, he has lots of visitors and his room is filled with flowers; by the fifth hospitalization, when his hope is

Dr. Michael Stein, associate professor of medicine at Brown University, believes that depression should be considered an opportunistic disease that accompanies HIV; that preexisting depression is a major factor in people engaging in behavior that exposes them to HIV and that postdiagnosis depression is a factor in infected people exposing others; that depression is a major factor in patients being noncompliant with their medications; and that untreated depression contributes directly to disease progression.

even more diminished and he needs extra support, the visitors may have dwindled and the flowers aren't there.

HIV positives fear or feel a sense of estrangement from community and healthy individuals, regarding themselves as outcasts or pariahs. These negative feelings stem from the double whammy of societal bias against people with disabilities and specifically stigmatization of people with AIDS. Perhaps in an attempt to lessen the blow, men with HIV often isolate themselves rather than expose themselves to rejection by others.

An aversion to those with HIV can be paralleled to the menstrual taboo, whereby women were once considered outcasts and even today aren't perceived as desirable sexual beings while menstruating. Early cultures were wary of females experiencing a monthly effusion of blood that sullied the whiteness of sheets and the purity of body and spirit. Although menstruation is part of a healthy woman's experience, it mimics disease through the pain, discomfort, and bleeding that in every other context signal injury, not health. Society writes a paradoxical script that dictates the definitions of health, illness, and cleanliness.

> **The double whammy of societal bias against people with disabilities and specifically stigmatization of people with AIDS causes some men with HIV to isolate themselves rather than expose themselves to rejection by others.**

Culture also restricts the sexual behavior of those who appear unhealthy. Even the natural process of birth is deemed to be unclean; the Catholic theologian St. Augustine wrote, "We are born between feces and urine." HIV-positive people, too, are considered untouchable.

Whereas menstruation creates the illusion of illness, asymptomatic HIV infection creates the illusion of health. Those who are asymptomatic become suspect in their outward presentation of health that does not signal "unclean" the way menstrual blood does. When others find someone is actually ill despite outward appearances, this can create a stigmatizing response that sets apart those who have broken this hygienic contract. This separation is even more severe than that imposed upon the modern menstruating woman. Being considered a pariah and the experience of isolation increases the desire to couple to rid oneself of loneliness. Social integration—becoming part of a community or a "family of choice" that validates one's identity as an HIV-positive individual, combined with incorporating that identity for oneself—will determine whether a person will become a viable member of a social group and be open to connecting with another individual. Lyons continues, "There is evidence that through even the most severe, life-threatening illness, social relationships can be preserved, effectively restructured, and even improved."[4]

Common Experience Creates a Shared Identity

Australia was established in 1788 as a penal colony (at Sydney) by the British. More than two hundred years later, this outpost for criminal outcasts has grown and evolved to become a country of 20 million people, proud of their shared national identity. Current estimates suggest that there are twice as many people with HIV worldwide as there are residents of Australia. Like the early Australians, HIV positives are considered outcasts. Rather than being grouped together on one continent, however, we are linked by our HIV status. How can positive people come together under one proud identity, as have the modern Aussies? What shifts must occur in our minds to transform us from outcasts to a cohesive group? One way is by choosing our own.

Shared Serostatus Relieves Dating Tension

Dating within the context of HIV may mean fishing in a different pond, either through self-selection or by restriction, whether this is perceived or real. And for some, dating/relationship options open up more postdiagnosis, since relationships are sometimes closer or more valued with the threat of their loss.

The shared experience of HIV may alleviate many of the "pre-existing," and sometimes uncomfortable, conditions of dating and beginning a relationship. Not having to worry about disclosure and rejection based on positive status eliminates this anxiety and fear. Dating is often a scary process if you have not conquered your fears about disclosure. It may even feel like your romantic life has ended. HIV often elicits feelings of sympathy and/or fear. Positives do not want their dates to see them as people to be pitied or avoided. Yet

when you feel as if you are
the only one who is positive
and, worse, believe no one
will want you, this often becomes a reality.

Independent of health status, the
frequency of male orgasms is influ-
enced most notably by age, with
men reaching their peak at age
thirty with 121 orgasms per year,
up from 104 at age twenty, declining to 84 per year by age forty,
and with 22 orgasms annually by
age seventy.[5]

Of course, if you are positive, you are most definitely
not the only one. As HIV
prevention efforts continue to
have limited success, the number of people who have posi-
tive status in common increases, which multiplies the chances of
finding empathy in a partner through shared experience. Also, as
people with HIV live longer, there will be increased opportunity to
develop skills to reenter the dating pool. Increased years of health
means increased years of being sexually active and/or able to perform, which potentially will increase the number of people with
HIV (see the box).

In its infancy, HIV within a single individual had a shorter lifespan that created self-limiting chances to spread the disease. That is
no longer the case. Now that people with HIV live a lot longer, the
chances of one positive person infecting more partners have increased. In fact, we need to acknowledge this lengthening of one's
sex life as a powerful emerging cofactor in increasing the spread of
HIV. Risk, as any good insurance agent will tell you, increases as
length of time exposed to it grows. Removing any and all social and
psychological factors, pure male physiology tells us that two years of
ejaculating is different from twelve or twenty.

**Condoms have acted as viral
stopwatches in the sprint that
was called the "gay cancer of
the eighties," when a person
was expected to live only
two years. Will these
stopwatches perform as well
in the marathon that is now
HIV?**

Every orgasm is a moment
in time, perhaps a more intense
or briefer moment than others,
but still a countable and measur-
able moment. Condoms have
acted as viral stopwatches in the
sprint that was called the "gay
cancer of the eighties," when
a person was expected to live
only two years. Will these stopwatches perform as well in the
marathon that is now HIV?

Shared serostatus relieves the tension of agonizing over whether we are acceptable—whether anyone will find us beautiful, or at least touchable. In 1939, a movie was released that featured cast members who were physically different, people who were assumed not to have sex lives, people who were literally and figuratively looked down on. Sixty years later the film is one of the best-loved movies of all time. It's *The Wizard of Oz,* and when these actors were brought from all over the country to play the Munchkins, the set suddenly became for many a big love feast. They couldn't keep their hands off each other. This may come as a surprise to those who would not expect midgets to have sex lives. Similarly, some don't expect HIV-positive people to be sexually active (or they perceive the HIV positive as overly sexual). While some may challenge the comparison of HIV-positive people to midgets, it allows us to explore how a commonality of difference can work as a magnetic force, drawing those who are "different" together.

> **A commonality of difference can work as a magnetic force, drawing those who are "different" together.**

Biology as Biography: Shared Stories

Those who share our biology share our biography—and can provide mutual support and understanding. Observing and socializing with others who join in our experiences allows us to use them as role models for successful adjustment. A unique and powerful synergy takes place when individuals with similar challenges can offer assistance to one another.

How this plays out with two positives can be demonstrated by the example of the "bartender." Sharing HIV can make one a better "bartender" to serve the complicated "cocktail" drug—the slang term for the protease inhibitor drugs that at times must be taken in combination with other drugs to work.

This "miracle" combination of drugs has been touted extensively in the press; however, there has been limited discussion on the role of the good "bartender"—someone there to say, "Are you ready for another?" or serve you "the usual." Whether your cocktail is a martini or a protease inhibitor, it is important to have someone there familiar with your cocktail needs and who knows when you would like a refill of your glass or prescription. As a partner to someone with HIV, you will often act as that bartender (or cocktail waitress, if you prefer).

As numbers of positives link up with each other, the stigma surrounding them shrinks. As positives meet a broader range of people with this common experience and challenge, their social circle shifts towards those whom they feel are accepting and more comfortable with them. Invariably it is harder to reject your own kind.

Rite of Passage

Sometimes the fear of contracting HIV, coupled with the sense of inevitability, sets the stage for a type of relief when you are diagnosed. It's almost like "Whew! Now that has happened, I can move on with my life." Diagnosis can then trigger change and evaluation of what is important in life, including romance.

Facing your own possible mortality can cause you to elevate the role of relationships in an increasingly meaningful way. Your time is allocated to those things that really matter.

Also, as we reach out to each other, we encounter people who have traveled the same road and say, "You are one of us now, and we'll show you how," and what is most important, "I understand." This empathy and mutual vulnerability can force (and speed up) intimacy. Though this immediate intimacy can sometimes work out, it is also something to be mindful of, especially if it feels awkward or uncomfortable for you.

Two Positives Can Equal Intensity

As we discussed in Chapter 3, how the partners perceive time will affect the rhythm of the relationship. Connecting with someone else who is positive when you were uncertain that love would ever be possible again has all the makings of a whirlwind romance. While some nonpositive couples will pull back when a budding relationship seems to be moving too fast, positive couples may be less hesitant and more likely to approach the beginning stages of coupling with vigor and exuberance. Maybe they are emboldened by the fact that they are living with HIV and not dying after all, or they are keenly aware that their own biological clock is ticking. Either way, positives may take higher leaps of faith and fall more deeply and quickly in love. But again, proceed with caution if the intimacy is on a fast track. You may run the risk of taking it too fast and too far, and get hurt in the end. On the other hand, this may be good and result in a deeper, more meaning-ful relationship than you would have had otherwise.

Proceed with caution if the intimacy is on a fast track.

Coupling with Positives for Negative Reasons

The support that an HIV-positive person can find in coupling with another positive can turn negative if the relationship is based al-most exclusively on HIV status. Some HIV-positive men believe that this relationship may be their last chance for romance, so they avoid certain conflicts and ignore incompatibilities out of fear that facing and dealing with them may end the romance, which could be their last chance for love. They also may be afraid that without their pri-mary caretaker, they are likely to get sicker. In my work with couples in therapy, specifically where at least one partner is positive, one of the more difficult questions to ask is "Would you be in this relation-ship if you weren't HIV positive?"

Psychiatrist and author Steven Schwartzberg, in his book *A Cri-sis of Meaning*, talks about how positives feel "tainted" and don't feel confident about finding new relationships. He quotes one positive man as saying: "In my relationship, it [HIV] has kept me from wan-dering, kept me more on the straight and narrow than I'm person-ally inclined to be. I feel the pressure to be this way, because (1) I'm infected, and I wouldn't want to be out there infecting other people, and (2) it would be hard to replace my current relationship with something more satisfying—after all, I'm damaged and damaging goods." Another positive patient stated, "Everyone has sympathy for people with [multiple sclerosis], people with cancer, people with any of a million other diseases. But to have a disease where the peo-ple are treated like pariahs . . . I feel tainted, bad blood."[6] A third in-terviewee was the most blunt when he said, "I don't think we'd still be together if it weren't for the [HIV]. . . . If the situation were dif-ferent, I would have ended things, we've had too many disagree-ments. . . . If we didn't have this to keep us together, it would have been easier to walk out."[7]

So how can a couple bravely assert their needs and move toward a resolution or even dissolution of a troubled relationship without believing, factually or otherwise, that this may impact their physical health? What are the stressors in a relationship, and how do we find an acceptable balance between need and independence?

Roberto is an outspoken, slim, HIV-positive, forty-four-year-old nurturing father of two. A higher leap of faith in a relationship with his partner, Terrence, has brought him both ecstasy and disappointment.

Roberto describes his initial "fairy tale" courtship with Terrence, their partial "falling out," and his current sense of urgency to stay committed to the relationship for fear of not finding another eligible HIV-positive male.

Listening to Roberto makes it clear that he believes preferring to couple with someone who is positive is a reasonable and good choice, but staying with that person—in a bad relationship—only because that person is positive isn't in his best interest.

Roberto is an active member of a support group for HIV-positive and HIV-negative individuals who are involved with positive people. According to Roberto, the support group is "full of people who feel locked into relationships with other positives." As he describes their relationships, "Those who were positive were afraid to venture out of the relationships because they were positive, and those who were negative felt obligated to take care of their partners who were positive."

The group members' tendencies seemed to mirror his own.

Roberto, a Mexican American disabled veteran, has been involved with Terrence, a bisexual, HIV-positive, African American male, for almost three years. He says what started out as a relationship of all-consuming love—two HIV-positive people sharing common ground, the trials and tribulations that come from having the disease, and the fight for their lives—has turned into something he has grown apart from but is still holding on to, partly for lack of better options.

Though Roberto describes himself and Terrence as "married," he has chosen to live apart from his partner, if only next door, and is trying to detach himself from a time when he was more dependent on him.

Roberto has progressed from living in an insulated HIV-positive world in which he looked to Terrence for stability and hope to a more independent place. Yet this new lack of closeness feels isolating and now at times frustrates him.

At the time of their first encounter Roberto had already shut himself off from the world after discovering he was HIV positive and had been misdiagnosed for eight years. He believes he contracted AIDS from unprotected sex he had in the U.S. Navy in the late 1980s, a time when he wasn't made aware of HIV. At the time he met Terrence, he was spending his days locked up inside a bedroom in his mother's house, away from his grown children and friends.

"After I found out I had AIDS, I retreated into my room; I thought I was going to die," Roberto said. "I had just lost a friend a year before to AIDS, and he shot dope; he was also a veteran. I didn't want to die like my friend; his family had turned their backs on him, treated him badly. I gave up on life, didn't want to have sex, felt unattractive, unloved, cursed, unwanted, ashamed."

Then he was introduced to Terrence, a dark-skinned, large, charismatic man. Roberto's sister had met him in a drug recovery support group. It was there where Terrence confessed that he was HIV positive.

"When I saw him, I said, 'Wow! I think I love him!' " Roberto exclaimed.

Terrence was also emerging from a time of isolation during which he had spent six years in jail for drug charges; during which time he became an advocate for others going through the same trials. He was released because of his HIV-positive status.

During their courtship Terrence pulled Roberto out of his shell, got him to come out publicly as HIV positive, and pushed him to start his volunteer career as an AIDS activist. Roberto came out to his entire family only a month after he was diagnosed correctly, on Father's Day, 1995. His family received the news well.

Terrence and Roberto soon moved into one apartment and "did everything together," which included volunteering at a local AIDS service organization where Terrence was a supervisor during the day, eating dinner together every night, and spending all their free time on the weekends with each other.

"He was the same age as me, had the same ideas, was very genuine," Roberto said. "We did everything together, we decided to take our medicine together after our T-cells started to drop, which translated into accepting the fact we both had AIDS, we went to the doctor together, and I didn't feel so all alone, he didn't feel so all alone. We were living exclusively in an HIV world. We made a pact we would end up dying together. We didn't know we would live."

Relationship tension came when Roberto, who had been opened up to the world of activism, became a spinning wheel of energy that couldn't stop. His independence is what he feels started the friction in his relationship with Terrence.

While he was living with Terrence, he took it upon himself to collect 500 signatures around his neighborhood for increased availability of HIV testing sites—a cause he couldn't part with after having been misdiagnosed for eight years and almost losing his life. In collecting the signatures, he came out as positive to all his neighbors in northwest Washington, DC—a very satisfying and liberating move.

"The secret was out. I felt really comfortable then," he said.

Roberto's latest community endeavor, since he has stopped living with Terrence, has been to start a social/support group for men who are HIV positive.

As time passed and Roberto became more and more involved in politics and the community, he felt less of a need for Terrence, who was climbing higher politically on a national level, to hold his hand as an activist or as an HIV-positive person.

"I've been let out of my cage, and I won't go back. It was professional rivalry. I didn't need for him to tell me what to do anymore. I'm not holding on to his coat tails so tight. I moved out to start my new life with HIV. I wasn't thinking anymore of dying with the virus, I was thinking about living with the virus," he said.

Lyons describes one's decreased dependence on a primary relationship and increased reliance on a broader social support system as "communal coping," where "couples, nuclear or extended family, or close friends may adopt the position that illness is 'our problem,' and so they cope with many of the emotional and instrumental aspects of a health problem together."[8]

Roberto developed this system of coping as a healthier way for him to deal with his illness. But though he and Terrence have grown apart, it is hard for Roberto to think about venturing outside the relationship for companionship. Roberto says now he and Terrence have a "close but distant relationship" in which they talk every day on the phone but don't see each other every day and rarely have sexual relations:

"We don't have a fairy tale relationship anymore. Reality is setting in. I live alone now. We are positive, we love each other. It's hard to find someone you love, who you are equal to in a lot of ways."

"We are growing apart, but I don't want to let go of him. There is no one else for me. There are not that many available men with HIV-positive status who don't look sickly. This leaves very few men for me. If I had some choices, I might be with someone else during the times we don't get along. We have different interests. I need to open my world up."

Roberto also said that partly he stays with Terrence because he is afraid of being alone, that "being HIV positive makes one more likely to want to be with someone. I don't want to die alone. I want someone to love me for who I am, Roberto who has AIDS, not feel pity or sorry for me."

Emotional Dumping Grounds: Use a Support Group, Not Your New Boyfriend

In situations like Roberto's, it is important to keep in mind the potential help a support group can provide for someone who is HIV positive. Roberto started and benefited from a support group late in his relationship with Terrence but could have benefited from one earlier on and might have avoided becoming overdependent in his relationship.

The fact that you are HIV positive can contribute to making you more physically and emotionally vulnerable. You are also vulnerable emotionally when first dating someone. Don't make yourself more emotionally exposed by using your date as an emotional dumping ground for all your feelings and fears about being positive. Especially don't do this during the very first stages of a relationship. Dumping emotions too early may force intimacy too quickly, something that often kills a budding relationship. And then you're left without a relationship and emotionally unprotected.

Dumping emotions too early may force intimacy too quickly, something that often kills a budding relationship.

To avoid this pitfall, find yourself an HIV-positive support group and/or a therapist versed in the subject of HIV. If your city or town has a local gay and lesbian community center (a list of gay community centers can be obtained at *www.gaycenter.org*), it will probably offer such a support

The U.S. national 800 number for the AIDS Counseling and Information Hotline is 1-800-590-2437, which can help you find organizations in your area.

group and a list of therapists: the groups are usually free, and the private therapy sessions are often prorated to suit your income (see the box). Also consult your gay community newspaper for HIV-related organizations that can point you in the right direction.

It may be a natural impulse to want to tell your *new* boyfriend everything you're feeling—a relief to have a special someone in which to confide. But holding back and sharing those tears and fears with professionals or a peer-led group is likely to be more emotionally healthy and appropriate. Peer groups and professionals can offer objectivity, frankness, and confrontation in a way that someone you're personally close to often cannot provide, for fear of hurting you or wanting to fix the problem right away, for example. Early on in a relationship it is not a good idea to reveal all, especially problems. Doing so is, again, rushing intimacy, and it may be perceived as a burden by your partner and backfire on the relationship. Good relationships need time to move into this kind of intimacy.

Sexual Infidelity: Can You Allow It?

Tibor, a vivacious, lanky, HIV-positive man originally from the Ukraine, is an HIV/AIDS educator within a close-knit Russian community. His story is also one of disillusionment from rushing into a relationship with someone simply because the other was positive.

"I met him in a bookstore café," Tibor begins. "We talked about our HIV status on the second date. You have lots of expectations with people when you are positive and they are positive. I thought getting involved with another positive person would enrich us both, that spiritually we could grow up together as a human beings. I was wrong. Some people are just sluts.

"He broke my heart. We were together six months. He left me in September [it was now December], but I still think about him about every day."

Tibor went on to describe how his ex moved into his apartment little by little, received calls on his beeper a lot, which was suspect, and one day Tibor went into a certain gay bar to play pool and discovered his lover in the bathroom with another guy.

"Some people are HIV-positive, but they don't want commitment. They don't care."

Coupling with Positives: Ethics or Self-Protection?

Fear of Infecting Negatives

Despite a lot of antigay, anti-HIV hype about irresponsible positive people anonymously infecting others, many positives say the guilt they would feel if they infected a negative person drowns out all desire to date from a negative pool. Surprisingly, this prejudice about positives being promiscuous comes not only from the heterosexual community but also from within the gay community. Another Schwartzberg interviewee stated, "There's the stereotype in the community that people who are positive were promiscuous, and there's a real judgmental attitude about that. . . . [I]t makes me angry that the gay community is so judgmental to their own people."[9]

So, contrary to popular belief, in addition to a way to decrease isolation, positives are choosing their own to prevent infecting others who don't have the disease.

While it may not be considered frequently by HIV prevention specialists, questions from a strictly epidemiological point of view include: How have HIV-positive people played a role—in their selection of sexual partners who are also positive—in slowing down the spread of infection? What would an HIV prevention campaign look like that recognizes that social phenomenon? If a segment of vegetarians chooses not to eat meat strictly for reasons of conscience, what percentage of the positive community select celibacy or dating within their own serostatus for similar altruistic reasons?

Many of the positive individuals interviewed for this book have stated that their reason for dating within their own serostatus is to be able to live with their own conscience. While this may be true, we must not discount the equally likely scenario that this is driven by a type of benevolence and genuine concern for their fellow man.

Louis, an energetic, wiry man with a twinkle in his eye, and Donald, a program analyst for a private environmental watchdog group, attend a regular monthly social for HIV-positive gay men.

Over appetizers and beer, they said they prefer to date HIV-positive people because, according to Louis, "It alleviates a lot of guilt. I would never have sex with someone who was negative without disclosing my status, but even if I were totally honest, if he turned positive after we had sex, I'd feel a lot of guilt about that. It could be my fault. Not knowing for sure wouldn't prevent me from feeling guilty."

Donald, who is happily involved with another positive male, also avoids the guilt of possible transmission. "I have problems dating negative people because I always have doubts and think I will in some way pass this on, and I would never forgive myself," he said. "I was involved with someone negative, and ended up thinking 'I can't go on like this.' That's the major reason I broke up with him. It was more of a problem with me, not him. I was so worried I might pass it on."

Roberto also fears infecting someone negative: "I think about going back to some guys I used to know, who say they don't care if I'm HIV positive. But I don't want to kiss them. I don't know if I'll infect them, but I'm more conscious of my infection. One slip to my friends and they could get infected. I don't want to be responsible for someone's death. If I don't date negative people, my conscience is clear."

Rejection from Negatives Turns Some toward Positives

Some positives choose to date other positives to avoid being rejected because of their own HIV status and the resulting psychological complications. A patient of mine once said, "I want the ability to feel secure without being responsible for others who are made uncomfortable with my status. My life would not have the same level of meaning, especially in the relationships with my peers and potential romantic interests, if our experiences in the world were too terribly different."

Relationships between positives, when based merely on a common fear of being rejected by negatives, are inherently unfulfilling, which people in this situation often come to realize. Such was the situation for Graham, whose heart had recently been crushed by someone (let's call him Trevor) who was also positive. He feels Trevor was using him for sex because Trevor's lover refused to sleep with him upon finding out he was positive. Graham, believing they had a connection beyond sex and regular trips to the pharmacy, wanted more. But although Graham was burned in this relationship, he will continue to date HIV-positive people in the future, to avoid the unbearable rejection he had experienced from an earlier, HIV-negative lover, based on serostatus.

> **Relationships between positives, when based merely on a common fear of being rejected by negatives, are inherently unfulfilling.**

Graham can forgive Trevor, the positive one who broke his heart, because he could relate to the rejection Trevor had felt from his lover. Again, empathy between two positives comes into play. "He told me he was positive right away, which immediately made me feel we had experiences in common," Graham says of his most recent lover. "I knew other guys that I found out about only through the grapevine. It might have been something Trevor and I shared. We could talk about it with each other. His leaving nearly destroyed me. I withdrew from everyone. I was as desperate and helpless as I've ever been in my life." But oddly, Graham isn't scared away from other positives and would choose to be rejected by a positive over his rejection by an earlier, negative lover who dumped him for being positive.

"I was in a relationship for ten years with someone who was negative, and when I turned positive, that was the end of it," Graham revealed. "He told my friends he hoped I would die a slow, painful death—when he was the one who had fooled around for ten years, while I fooled around only once. After that I haven't dated any negative people," he adds bitterly. "I'm looking for someone positive, because it solves a lot of problems. Often, the negative one will use your positive status against you in an argument, and I know how much that can sting. The one I was with for ten years did that to me. Someone who's negative can't empathize, because he's never been there. For instance, if you're tired, under the weather, other positives can know what that feels like. They will understand why you don't want to go dancing. They don't hold it against you, don't make you feel like a disappointment to them."

Others who are positive confirm Graham's fears of rejection by those who don't share their illness. Tibor also chooses to date positives, even in the face of his recent "dumping" by another positive man: "I prefer to date HIV-positive people because we can grow up together, take care of each other, help with medications, cope and pray together, learn from each other, and love. I was rejected by two guys because of my HIV status. One guy admitted outright that he was terrified, while the other took the cowardly way out—he said he'd call and never did."

Protecting Ourselves from Negative Reactions

Dawson is a 45-year-old retiree from Wall Street. He frequents the gym and has the chest to prove it. He has lived with HIV for more than a decade and feels he has experienced bias against him for being positive, and therefore immediately discloses his HIV status to a potential date. He is currently dating his third positive boyfriend and had a bad romantic experience with someone negative as well:

"I had a relationship with a negative person for four years, and we fought constantly. He would ask why the *Advocate* writes all these articles about positive people and never writes about the negative people and the suffering they go through. He had problems too, he claimed. I broke up with him, and I never heard from him again. He never checked up on me.

"I didn't tell him I was positive for the first two months of our relationship, though we had protected sex. He was angry and said he wouldn't have fallen in love with me had he known. Before I thought my partner needed to get a chance to know me as a person. Now I know that to know me as a person is knowing this large part of me, and I'll disclose [my status] right away."

Now Dawson says, "I prefer not to date negatives at all. In fact, I even prefer HIV-positive friends. That way they don't judge you. I'm very careful about who my friends are."

Dawson appears to feel that even when someone who is negative tries to be supportive, the effort can lack genuine empathy. This offering of assistance and the wish to be helpful is countered by his awareness of a "one up" perspective. He feels someone whose health situation is not certain or is in jeopardy cannot understand fully what he and others like him are going through. The response that Dawson may receive is out of synch with what he needs and may be too supportive at times and insufficient at others: his illness acts like a language that separates him from others who can't speak it no matter how hard they try; the accent is still apparent.

Discordance among Positives

The challenges faced by serodiscordant couples discussed in Chapter 3 affect positive couples as well. Partners can share the same serostatus but have different experiences with the disease. When one partner, for example, has 700 T-cells and the other has 70 or 7, the disparity in medical stability can play out in shifting expectations, roles, and the balance of power. One partner may be dealing with loss of independence, money, sexual ability, and physical energy or just the general psychological and physical fallout from long-term survival, whereas the other is wrestling with the crisis of recent diagnosis or reaping the benefit of a more hopeful medical outcome.

How the problems affect the individuals involved and the relationship can vary tremendously and are not always predictable or logical. The partner with 700 T-cells may experience anticipatory survivor guilt or end up ashamed from feeling resentful of caretaking for which he feels obligated. The partner with many fewer T-cells may tire over an extended period of the beneficence of the healthier partner who gives and gives. Loving partners may find their empathy for their shared plight challenged along with their vows to stand by each other till the end. There is the risk of anger becoming an underlying emotion in a home shared by positives who are at different stages of their disease.

> **When one partner has 700 T-cells and the other has 70 or 7, the disparity in medical stability can play out in shifting expectations, roles, and the balance of power.**

In the past, health care efforts were trained almost exclusively on the member of a couple identified as the primary patient, but now providers are beginning to respond as well to the negative effects—psychological as well as physical—on the primary caregiving partner. Increased stress and compromised health are of particular concern when the caregiver is also positive. If you and your partner are both positive, you may be able to craft the life together that you envisioned if you think ahead about how you'll deal with common problems so as to preserve health—your own, your partner's, and your relationship's.

Care: For Yourself and Each Other

The supportive role we play for our partners can have negative implications for those of us who act as the primary caregiver. You'll need to monitor how this plays out physically or emotionally in your lives. Be sure to give yourself permission to take some healing time as well. Accept early on that your receipt of care and nurturance can help prevent you from experiencing a premature burnout that can manifest itself in a variety of ways: exhaustion, anger, resentment or emotional withdrawal. In contrast, receiving care from someone more healthy can also create stress and feelings of guilt for the recipient, which contributes to a type of discordance as well. Thus, having a balanced plan brings greater harmony to the relationship.

HIV-positive couples must deal with many of the same challenges and questions faced by elderly couples. Confusion and concern over health, medications, and views and discussions (or avoidance) of their own mortality are woven into the tapestry of the couple's lives. Questions such as "Who will survive?" and "Will we each have enough strength for caretaking when we're both suffering fragile health?" are always in the background. Bringing these challenges into the foreground and addressing them, especially as the disease has become chronic, will pave the way to having both confidence and experience when and if the illness turns more acute.

Ways to address these discordancy challenges could include the following:

- Join your partner's doctor appointments. Weave health and the preservation of it into your daily lives.
- Recognize the value of "stress inoculation," defined as being exposed repeatedly to low levels of stress as a way to eventually face or be immunized against a larger problem. An example would be the first time you experience a medication side effect and the doctor solves the problem with a different dose. A series of these small successes will succeed in making you both stronger in facing the illness.
- Make use of the unanticipated benefits of illness, like extra time for family, friends, and travel. This will allow you to prioritize your values, such as focusing on yourself and your relationship, not just on your careers (as men have been socialized to do). By doing so you'll strengthen the ties you have as a couple and move to a greater intimacy.

Jimmy and Peter: Same Status, Different Views

The issue of difference came up while I was talking to Jimmy and Peter, a young, positive couple, together not quite two years, who met through Jimmy's personals ad for an "HIV-positive partner." Though both are currently medically stable and happy together, they differ in how they are dealing with their illness. The disparity in their acceptance of the illness parallels their respective commitment to the relationship.

Jimmy has known he was HIV-positive for eight years, is retired due to HIV, is proactive about his treatment, and says he "feels married to Peter," with whom he has lived for more than a year.

Peter, on the other hand, though he has been diagnosed for six years, is closeted about his serostatus, especially at work, knows his pills only by color, can't imagine a time when either one of them may approach a premature death, and feels as if he and Jimmy are at the "boyfriends" as opposed to "marriage" stage. Both look completely healthy. As a couple, they don't have powers of attorney, and neither has a will.

They live in homey suburban duplex outside of Denver, with lots of plants and comfortable furniture. Jimmy stands over six feet tall, is blond, brown-eyed, and twenty-eight-years old. He was diagnosed at age twenty-one but thinks he contracted HIV when he was seventeen. He's had to make a career change because of his past health failings—he retired from physical therapy, a stressful and physical profession—and is attending a community college for a business degree while he lives off his disability checks. Until he had to quit his job, he was pretty closeted about his positive status. Now he resents hiding it. Jimmy is extremely verbal, openly committed to Peter, and has convinced Peter to attend couples' therapy so that "they can communicate better and strengthen their relationship."

Peter, at age twenty-nine, is shy, possesses a quiet candor, and though happily involved with Jimmy, is hesitant to use the word "marriage" when describing their relationship. In our interview, this fact surprises Jimmy. Peter is also attempting a career switch, from occupational therapist to computer programmer, but says the switch is not related to his HIV status.

When asked if they expect to be present when the other dies, Peter says he hasn't thought about it and "is scared of being a caregiver" and is "equally reluctant to let someone else take control." In contrast, Jimmy says he has thought about the grim prospect and would feel totally comfortable being Peter's caregiver. "I probably have had HIV longer than Peter, am more drug resistant, so there are more chances I'd get sick," he said. He feels that Peter would also make a good caregiver, despite Peter's hesitance. So their different views, which are perfectly normal for any couple while not causing a major problem in their relationship thus far, could change should either fall ill—though Jimmy describes Peter as "not a deserter."

When One Is More Ill

Mutual support between two positives can be stretched thin whether the disparity is in health status or in their commitment to health care. At those times the one who is more "well" or is taking steps to stay well can feel overwhelmed. This leads to fears perhaps of becoming a premature caregiver or experiencing a more sudden loss, which often triggers frustration and anger with the partner. Sometimes the fact that both people are positive is just plain challenging.

Mitch is a swarthy, muscular orthopedist at a Connecticut university hospital. His baldness makes his thick mustache and sex appeal stand out that much more. Mitch recently lost his lover, Robert, to complications associated with AIDS. Mitch says he was devastated. "It's hard for two positives to support themselves, because they both need help," he said. "It depends on where they are in their own acceptance of living with HIV."

Accepting Help

For those who place a high value on being independent and self-reliant, receiving someone else's care may provoke responses ranging from awkwardness to anger. This uneasiness may not be immediately apparent, because couples will exert energy in creating and maintaining optimism during initial hospitalizations. It is when these roles become more predictive due to repeated encounters with the health care system that readjustments have to be made. These changes may test the ability of a couple to adapt to these new roles. In extreme cases, the more ill partner, facing fears of becoming a burden, may even attempt to separate from his companion in his own altruistic attempt to protect him.

Donald, involved in a new long-distance relationship, says he has trouble accepting help and would consequently have a harder time if he was the one who became ill first: "I know that if my partner were dying it would bother me, but I would be there till the end. But if I were sick first, it would drive me insane that I was holding him back. It would make me feel guilty. I do everything myself anyway. I've always been that way. I would have to adjust if I really needed someone. A true friend is someone who comes to you when you're dying and wipes your ass." While Donald acknowledges his problem in accepting help, he contrasts that with his final statement and the realization of the need for assistance in what will be his most vulnerable moments.

A major factor leading to the end of Tibor's most recent relationship was his lover's inability to accept care. "I was concerned about his health more than mine," Tibor said. "He didn't take care of himself. He wasn't taking his medication properly. I'm not going to be someone's case manager; I'm supposed to be his boyfriend. It needs to be fifty/fifty."

How *do* positive partners take care of each other and the relationship? In response, Lyons and colleagues once again emphasize that one must assume a good "communal or relationship approach to coping . . . and we must ask, 'What is it that people with disabling health problems and their significant others need from each other to facilitate coping and adaptation?' "[10]

When one's partner experiences a progression of the disease, the healthier one may see his own fears actualized. The ill partner may, however, also act as a role model by showing that illness can be navigated with grace. On the other hand, the increasing emotional needs and the creation of protective distance between partners can contribute to disharmony in a basically caring relationship.

Facing Problems Together

I often explore the partners' history in facing adversity in my work with couples. What was the couples' prior experience in facing life stressors conjointly, such as infidelity, job loss, death of a family member, or financial difficulties? The ability to succeed or feel like a team in facing these challenges will be a frame of reference for the upcoming challenges HIV may bring.

Care for the Caregiver

When we partner with positive people, invariably we are concerned with how our health impacts the health of our partners. Among the many thoughts pertaining to illness and relationships that I ask the couple to consider are "Who takes care of the caregiver?" and "What steps are put in place to do this?" Ways in which successful couples clear this hurdle include the following:

- Reach out and formulate support systems—whether through friends, professional organizations, or therapy.
- Create healing time and space for each other. This may involve allowing time away from each other—whether you do this with a weekend retreat or by using the guest bedroom down the hall when you know you will be up all night not feeling well and don't want to wake your partner.
- Have someone as a touchstone. I encourage each partner to use this person as a reference point outside the relationship with whom to discuss important issues. I have often invited these third parties into our therapy sessions when we face an impasse and I need their valuable and often *expert* opinion on what is going on with the couple.

Sharing a Support System

Also, in what way will partners access the same support? I shared with my positive partner the same physician, massage therapist, and hairdresser, but I also have benefited from his other caregivers. Once I spent the whole day crying at my office, convinced that the dark splotches I had recently discovered on my skin were Kaposi's sarcoma lesions The soonest I could set up an appointment with a dermatologist was three weeks away. My partner had an appointment with his skin specialist scheduled for that very afternoon. With Jerry's consent, I decided to join my lover's appointment. After hiking up my pants and exposing my "lesions," I was greatly relieved when the doctor pointed at the spots and intoned in a rather routine voice, "bug bite, bug bite, bug bite." Sometimes even a hypochondriac like me (I know—a bad combination with an incurable illness) has to just look back at things and laugh, realizing I have had occasional problems before I turned positive and am probably going to keep having them.

How we nurture ourselves and allow ourselves to be nurtured is an integral part of the healing process. Certainly we should expect some of this nuturing in our relationships.

When two people are immunologically compromised, the fragility or strength of their immune system can have direct consequences on their partner's health. It may not be unusual for a partner to say "Can you scratch my back?" But the other may feel, "If I scratch his back, I may catch (under my fingernails) whatever it is that is making his back itchy." The experience of being positive conditions responses in a variety of ways, and small, simple requests that arise in a relationship can become cause for anxiety and misunderstanding.

How we nurture ourselves and allow ourselves to be nurtured is an integral part of the healing process.

This requires increased creativity in expressing intimacy. Intimacy based on candor and safety would allow us to respond, "I really want to scratch your back, but until you clear up this rash, I can't. Just know I still love you." Having a wooden backscratcher or lotion and gloves handy is also a good idea.

It is some people's view and my clinical belief that if other aspects of the relationship are healthy and intact, the benefits of coupling and the life-extending and enriching promise of the relationship have a clear medical and psychological benefit to the immune system. I know very few people who would prefer to live like the main character in the TV movie *The Boy in the Plastic Bubble,* who had to be protected from all the germs in the world and lived in a specially constructed isolation tent, all the while aching for human contact.

Different Perceptions of Risk

The next two sections discuss bareback sex (sex without a condom) and the viral elite (those with a low viral load because they have access to medication)—two new factors to consider when it comes to being physically intimate with HIV-positive men. The first is a sexual practice perceived to be of low risk, given the individuals' HIV status; the second is a health status that is also perceived as low risk. Both perceptions of lower risk may be true in some circumstances, but the jury is still out. Researchers and the HIV community are still debating the health risks of barebacking and the transmission risks for someone with a low viral load. Remember, the virus cannot be inactivated and is highly mutagenic, and anal intercourse can cause abrasions that compromise the rectal lining and thus facilitate transmission. You need to be aware that real risks remain.

The New Sexual Liberation: Bareback Sex

A trend frequently mentioned in personal ads and Internet chat rooms and even specialized house parties, bareback sex signifies the latest form of sexual liberation. "Distinct from an infrequent [slipup], drunken mishap, or safer-sex 'relapse,' barebacking represents a conscious, firm decision to forgo condoms and, despite the dangers, unapologetically revel in the pleasure of doing it raw," writes Michael Scarce, author and prevention educator.[11] This phenomenon occurs frequently with one positive person dating another exercising the option of "bareback," or "raw" sex—when a couple forgoes condoms, given the fact that both are already infected.

But of course there is a hitch, or a possible price to pay—the chance of reinfection, a risk that was only recently brought to the forefront, which has been debated by scientists but nonetheless looms as a serious possible threat. Reinfection occurs when someone with one strain of HIV develops an additional strain or more of the same strain from a partner who is infected.

Bareback sex opponents say the longer people stay on anti-HIV therapy, the more vulnerable they might be to reinfection with a drug-resistant strain. For those who are treatment naïve (those who have never been prescribed medication before), once they do decide to pursue treatment, prescribing options may be more limited due to their exposure to this drug-resistant strain, in effect creating what is known as a "superinfection," which is much harder to combat. Those in the public health field also note that barebacking increases the possibility of contracting other STDs,

The *New England Journal of Medicine* published a letter suggesting that protease inhibitors have "altered the perception of risk" of contracting HIV for many gay men and that 26 percent of the men surveyed reported being "less concerned" about becoming HIV positive because of the new treatments, and "15 percent had already had unprotected anal sex because of their decreased concern."[12]

which would be devastating to a compromised immune system. Finally, they mention that possible funding cuts for HIV prevention could occur if "raw sex" gets full-scale media attention. (The risks of barebacking for negative-negative couples is discussed in Chapter 5.)

Men choose barebacking for various reasons. It has been suggested that the phenomenon may be linked to the perceived effectiveness of protease inhibitors and the promise of "morning after" exposure treatment, a cocktail of drugs taken the day after possible exposure, which supposedly kills the virus (this treatment was discussed in Chapter 3). Others engaging in the practice say they just want their lives and their bodies back, after a couple of decades of sexual inhibitions caused by the disease. They wish to make the most of whatever life they have left, which includes sexual pleasure, despite the documented risk to the health of both (see the box).

Jimmy and Peter, both positive, fall into the latter category. They made the choice not to use condoms after Jimmy broached the subject after a couple of dates, and they continue this practice with each other. They will don condoms when, on occasion, they bring a third party into their bed.

"Before the first time we had sex, we talked about it," Jimmy said with great ease and confidence. "It felt like we would be dating for a while. I'm not convinced of the chance of reinfection. When I was with my former lover, I enjoyed not using a condom. . . . It was a risk I was happy to take."

For Peter, bareback sex is a new experience. "Not using condoms was new to me. I was a little worried; it didn't feel right. I've been told by everyone to use condoms," he said.

Some men who choose barebacking say they just want their lives and their bodies back, after a couple of decades of sexual inhibitions caused by the disease.

Jimmy continued, "Condoms represent so many things. . . . The lack of a condom brings intimacy. . . . If I were to trick with someone positive, it wouldn't be appropriate to bareback; I wouldn't want to be that close. But if bareback sex means reinfection, then Peter and I would eventually have identical strains of HIV. Then we could buy our drugs in bulk," Jimmy said with a laugh. "By not wearing a condom we refuse to be limited in our sexual expression. It's empowering not to use a condom," he concluded (see the box).

Marc Ebenhoch, a young ex-marine, was quoted in the *New York Times Magazine* as saying "In a way, it's a relief. I don't have to wonder anymore. That awful waiting is gone. So now, if I do find someone, the relationship can be 100 percent real with nothing in the way. That's what I want: 100 percent natural, wholesome and real. Maybe now that I'm [HIV positive], I can finally have my life."[14]

IAN: RAISED IN THE "OLD SCHOOL"

Ian is another who engaged in bareback sex. Now deceased, when we met he was working on achieving both a Buddha frame of mind and a Buddha body, though he also said he was trying to lose weight and complained about a bit of a "protease paunch" (a common side effect of his medicine, which causes fat to redistribute toward his middle). He was a former socialite and disco baby who now donned a baseball cap and a blazer with art sewn on the back. After a disastrous love affair with someone who took him for a ride (leaving him for a rich lawyer), he was living on his $475-a-month disability check and the generosity of friends. People remembered when he was wealthy and shared. Now he lived rent-free with a friend who was dying of cancer, received tickets from his "ticket goddess," got invited to din-

The *Bay Area Reporter* highlighted the results of a survey, conducted primarily in San Francisco's Castro district in March 1998. Of 105 men who have sex with men, 37 percent had had unprotected anal sex during the previous six months. This was a follow-up survey to one conducted by ACT UP/Golden Gate, in 1994. At that time, according to the report, 24 percent reported engaging in unprotected anal sex.[13] This was a significant increase that followed the mass availability of and early optimism surrounding these new drugs.

ner by friends, and attended free art shows and music perfor-
mances.

He had the remnants of Kaposi's sarcoma on his face and a lot
of humor. "If you had seen me two months ago, I looked like *101
Dalmatians* meets Barney!" he joked, raising what chemotherapy
has left of his eyebrows.

Ian grew up in old school, old-money Santa Barbara, and his
"Mama didn't raise no punk." He opened the doors for ladies of all
kinds. Ian was cultured. He sent thank you notes and used the
proper forks, knew which wines went with what foods, knew what
to look for in the ballet, and could deconstruct modern art.

Part of that culture included caring for the "great unwashed." It
did not include eating or traveling with them. His was the perfect
upper-middle-class life, at least in appearance, which so often is
more important as well as more photogenic than the truth. His family was a "good family," well respected in the community. They sum-
mered on the shore, had Bloody Mary brunches, cocktail hours,
and proper dinners. Topics of conversation did not include his father's marital indiscretions, his sister's heroin habit, or Ian having
sex with the neighbor boy. All of which were acceptable, if kept
quiet, except for Ian being gay. He characterized himself as the pink
sheep of the family, his father as Darth Vader, and his siblings as
terrible and horrible.

Ian was looking for a husband: "I don't want to be a daddy. I
want one for myself." He wants someone like him, able to move
from black tie circles to rather kinky circles. "The only problem
with that is that they are all dead," he said, hands raised in exasper-
ation. He reassured himself, "I'm sure there is somebody out there
for me. I'm just hoping he's not in Chicago."

Ian was moving in the right circles to find a husband, but he already knew everyone, and the ones that were in his league were out
of the running. For his soul, he counseled prisoners and homeless
people with HIV. He joined boards and councils to find a husband.

His being a long-term survivor had affected his search for love.
He was also diagnosed under unique circumstances. In 1984, as a
medical student, working at the Massachusetts Institute of Technol-
ogy, he signed up for a study being conducted by Dr. David Ho. After having provided several blood and semen specimens, he started
hearing news reports about the study finding HTLV (human T-cell
lymphotropic virus, now called HIV) in the semen sample of a

healthy twenty-nine-year-old male. Sitting in the lunchroom at MIT watching the news, he started to wonder, "There are only fifty people in the study." He finally called a friend involved in the research and asked, "Is that ME?" The friend replied, "Didn't anybody tell you?"

"So now I'm sitting here with a loaded gun. It doesn't do anything for your sex drive, I'll tell you that."

Ian had gone from prince to pauper. He had survived several eras and had the artifacts to prove it: a macramé belt from the early 1970s, which he wore to Egypt with his strawberry blonde hair in a ponytail (something the Egyptian naval officers found attractive). During the disco age he found the great love of his life in New York, then designed laser light shows for Muammar al-Qaddafi of Libya, and did drugs with a variety of celebrities. Penthouses, beach houses, cocaine and wine, the Limelight disco, the A-list: this was Ian's element.

Because he thought of his penis as a potential harbinger of death, he dated only HIV-positive men. He tried to date HIV-negative men, but he was so worried he would not go beyond a certain point sexually. Having said that, he also did not believe in condoms.

Though he had been through a battle and seen better times as a long-time survivor diagnosed in 1984, when we talked he was holding a "live for the moment" attitude.

"If I were to start to worry about viral strains, I might as well roll over and play dead," he exclaimed. Since he didn't know how long he had on this earth anyway, he said, he wanted to have fun while he was here. If he were to start to ruminate, that itself would be a kind of death. Sadly, Ian died a year after our interview. Hundreds of friends attended his memorial service.

BAREBACKING: REBELLION, GIFT, OR ACCEPTABLE RISK?

Others echo the following sentiment: "The attention focused on anal sex as a risk activity has given it even more symbolic meaning as an act of profound intimacy or even rebellion. . . . [B]arebacking can thus be seen as merely the latest in a long line of challenges by gay men to the sexual status quo and the institutions which support it . . . a small, but cherished compensation for having HIV."[15]

There are different degrees and choices to be made concerning bareback sex. A couple may not engage in it at all—and decide to use condoms or not engage in anal or oral intercourse. A couple may decide not to use condoms and risk reinfection. Or a couple can decide not to use condoms but try to withdraw the penis from the anus or mouth before ejaculation.

Positives, and those who have sex with us, cover the entire spectrum of attitudes and practices—from "bug chasers," who desire infection and often advertise on the Internet, calling HIV "the gift,"[16] to those who are completely repulsed by the idea of putting themselves at further risk. The following examples exhibit different degrees of caution regarding bareback sex.

Mitch and his partner stopped engaging in anal sex altogether and never ejaculate into each other's mouths. Mitch feels that participating in bareback sex is a personal choice but "really hopes people understand there is a risk of reinfection."

Louis also "doesn't see anything wrong with bareback sex. . . . It is a personal choice between those two people," he said. "But I believe in reinfection. It is adding more virus to your system after you take drugs getting it out of your system. It is self-defeating. I would want my partner to pull out before he came."

Donald says that he engages in bareback sex with his current partner but withdraws before they ejaculate, and they have agreed between them to cease engaging in bareback sex if one or the other goes outside the relationship for sex.

By contrast, Dawson says that he and his partner never liked anal intercourse, but if they did, they would definitely use condoms.

"It's a guilt issue," Dawson said. "I'm not going to worry, because I'm practicing safe sex."

Stephen Follansbee of Castro's Infectious Disease Medical Group puts it differently: "Until we understand what is protective immunity regarding HIV, it's cavalier to think 'once infected, never reinfected.' "[17]

The Viral Elite

Though Ian practiced bareback sex, he also stated his desire to date only men with "over 250 T-cells." After having considered himself lethal for many years, he was starting to look at his prospective lovers as potential health hazards as opposed to the other way around. He used to worry about infecting others; now that he was dating only HIV-positive men, he worried about the viral load of his lovers. In other words, because his immune system was compromised, what did these folks have that he did not have and could catch?

This creates a viral hierarchy of both desirability and acceptability based on the accuracy of lab tests and how "sick" we look.

How "undesirable" we look is not necessarily a unique view within the HIV community. It is just as easy to fill in the same statement with "how 'black' one looks" in determining access to broadening avenues of power and choice, whether it be in sexual/romantic partner choices or political power.

Latinos and African Americans who climb the highest in the power elite tend to be lighter skinned than other members of their own racial group. As Colin Powell explained to Henry Louis Gates, Jr., in *The New Yorker* when questioned about his popularity among whites, "Thing is, I ain't that black."[18]

How black or how sick we look will correlate to the amount of stigma we face both within our group and without.

Our ability to "pass" like the octaroons and quadroons of New Orleans (people who possessed one-eighth or one-fourth black blood and were significantly fairer in complexion) has been a keen skill many gays and lesbians who remain in the closet to varying degrees developed to survive in a heterosexual-dominated world. Your ability to maintain your health or purity of blood and the appearance of it will determine your access to the executive rest room or, as the case may be, bedroom. If you are not out about your own status, being partnered with someone who is visibly ill, tired, thin, or pale moves the spotlight closer and may "out" you sooner than you'd planned.

And, of course, a prospective partner's viral load brings up the inevitable questions about how the other person's health will factor into your own. Will you choose a relationship with someone whose immune functioning is worse than yours if it could further compromise your health status? Does love conquer all? Is it the magic bullet that we once believed penicillin to be? If the other person is more ill than you, who will take care of you?

> **Your ability to maintain your health or purity of blood and the appearance of it will determine your access to the executive rest room or, as the case may be, bedroom.**

Five Signs of a Healthy Mature Relationship

Even though having a positive partner bestows on us shared experience and possibly increased intimacy, security, and mutual empathy, we have many hurdles to clear as HIV-positive couples. None of these necessarily preclude us from having fulfilling relationships, however. Couples who aspire to the following attributes, whether the partners are both HIV-positive, both negative, or serodiscordant, stand a good chance of having healthy mature relationships:

- Inner strength and solid sense of identity; a willingness to expose your innermost self while being strong enough to be vulnerable
- A full acceptance of the other as he is, without the need to manipulate and control
- Each receiving by giving to the other and becoming greater for the act of giving
- A recognition that a lasting relationship is often a process in which passion abundantly present at the onset is transformed into intimacy and commitment, more enduring qualities, which then sustain the relationship
- Nurturing, protecting, and caring; wanting to be together as opposed to needing to be together

Incurable Romantics: Ted and Joel

For one couple, the navigation of HIV seems to be a clear, honest journey.

Etch-A-Sketch, windup trains, a bright red ball, and silver jacks—this row house, like those of many of its neighbors in Brooklyn Heights, is cluttered with toys. But Ted and Joel, both thirty-eight, have things to worry about beyond mortgages, potholes, and available parking spaces.

Their attraction for each other goes beyond the obvious signs one looks for in a mate. Ted is a government official whose hazel eyes are framed by glasses popular with poets and artists of an earlier beat generation.

"He was a red flag man. All my red flags went off the first time

I saw Joel," Ted states as he strokes the hair on the bottom of his chin. Ted is olive-skinned with his roots in the Mediterranean. Joel is a light-skinned black man who possesses a languid sensuality, tall, lean with loose curly hair not long enough to be mistaken for that of a Rastafarian.

Dark tortoiseshell glasses are what Ted removes to rub his eyes, red from reading too many reports. Joel, you would imagine, probably didn't remove his seashell necklace during his last period of exertion, whether it was bicycling through a park or making love.

They first met in the halls of the Senate. Both went to Washington to lobby for the authorization of the Ryan White Comprehensive AIDS Research Emergency (CARE) Act of 1990 to increase funding for people with AIDS.

Ted, who at times still works seven days a week, states, "All my relationships have suffered because of work." Contemplating one possible future, he adds, "My goal when we moved to New York was to have a good enough résumé so it could be read at my wake."

When he met Ted, Joel was "working overtime" as well to ensure a kind of different future. "I was dating four people at the same time. . . . I was determined," he paused with some hesitation. "My first fear was I would never have a relationship. I figured no one would want an HIV-positive nigger."

Joel, who was diagnosed positive in the winter of 1992, says, "After that, I always knew I wanted to date someone else positive."

Ted, who believes he was infected while he was a seminary student, learned the results "November 14, 1989, at 4:00 P.M. It was between meetings."

As he recalls that with clarity, I can't help reflecting on the day in late September 1993 when I found out that I was positive. The exact date, unlike Ted's, escapes me, but the sorrowful look in the brown eyes of the health clinic counselor who told me does not.

When asked about the Catholic church's expectation of chastity, Ted smiles and replies, "Little did I know I was going into a bathhouse where you take vows."

Then, like a scene from a shuffleboard game in a Miami retirement center, we switch to talking about our medications and then back to men. "I'm on the cocktail," Joel says, while I nod in agreement, being on a similar regimen myself. Ted says he's not on the regimen because he has "naturally occurring low viral load and high T-cells."

Perhaps the one reason he prefers positive partners, Ted continues, is "they just don't understand," referring to those who are HIV negative. "One time I lost 800 T-cells—from over 1,300 to 460." Ted then goes on to describe the amount of energy he expends on "a type of reverse or inverted caregiving to reassure the negative people around me that I'm well." He was echoing the theme that many positive people have brought up to me—the question of whether, when people ask us how we are doing, we answer politely, "Fine, and you?" or give them the latest lab results.

Shifting your responses depending on how you believe they will be taken can be tiresome. Will the other person respond in a worried, overreactive manner that may require a minicourse in immunology or with a cool nonchalance when you were hoping for some warmth and support? Once again, this is an area where having a shared experience and understanding may make things easier. The application of the Golden Rule is always easier the more similar the "others" are to you.

Joel and Ted chime in simultaneously when asked about their concerns for their relationship if their diseases progress. "I hate to be taken care of," Ted says, then adds, "If he ever died on me. . . . I would break his neck and kill him." He later adds, "I was taught that being sick was a sign of weakness."

Joel offers in a lower and uncertain voice, "I don't know how that will be." Whereas they both admit to having a fatalistic outlook about their shared disease, they have a sense of optimism and perhaps believe that for now that question doesn't need to be answered.

The challenges they face are perhaps more common to the struggles many gay men face when defining roles. An example is getting Ted to slow down and relax: "I had my first vacation with Joel that was not attributed to a friend dying." So whereas many doctors may have advised him to reduce stress, it wasn't until he was coupled with Joel that this occurred. Living a compressed life can create this urgent desire to accomplish. The urgency can lead to shortened life and perhaps a lengthier obituary. Working with people with HIV often involves encouraging them to allow and aggressively pursue joy and to permit themselves to be nurtured.

Joel cleans the house, Ted writes him poetry, and both bring home the toys scattered around the house. How they define play is extended into other areas as well: "I heard from a friend, before I slept with Ted, that he liked to have bareback sex, which intrigued me." They don't practice monogamy and state that their "goal is emotional fidelity" and they "don't do it in the house." Expanding on the rules of their relationship, they stress the importance of "being honest and forthcoming," adding, "The trust we develop is because we are active in creating it." This last rule they shared with me had a freshness to it since they had canceled an earlier interview because of "relationship problems," and perhaps trust was one of the issues they needed to work out.

"The challenge has been being forthright while not being monogamous." Ted adds, "It's not to dethrill the experience of outside sex. In some ways it is trickier because I'm so attracted to Joel."

Asked in what ways have they solidified their relationship that allows this flexibility, Ted says, "On the Brooklyn Bridge we exchanged rings last September," and "I told Joel 'I want you to have this forever, and I want it back only if you break my heart.' "

Asked for some closing thoughts that they have for one another and their relationship, Ted answered first, with both warmth and confidence: "I can't imagine living without Joel. Even when we were going through this last difficult time, I couldn't hate him the way I wanted to."

Joel says his feeling for Ted includes "Admiration, for someone who is always trying to do the right thing. . . . He is my hero, my absolute hero, and living with him is amazing."

FIVE

JUMPER CABLES
AND RELATIONSHIPS
Negatives with Negatives

MARK E. WOJCIK[1]

I am HIV negative, and my boyfriend of the last nine years is also negative. Even so, AIDS brought us together. We met at the Tenth International Conference on AIDS in Yokohama, Japan, where I was giving a speech on AIDS discrimination by funeral homes[2] and he was representing southern Europe as a delegate from the European Council of AIDS Service Organizations (EuroCASO). I assumed that he was positive; he assumed that I was positive. I do not remember whether we corrected those assumptions before we left Japan or when we met later the following month in Italy. I only remember that I was in love with someone who was loving and wonderful. HIV would complicate things, but it would not stop me from entering a new relationship with him.

My earlier relationships had been with men who were HIV positive. Eddie, for one, was a handsome Latino I met at an art gallery opening in Chelsea, New York. He did not tell me that he was positive until we had been dating (and having sex) for two months. The moment of disclosure was obviously difficult for him—made more difficult by the fact that he had not told me about his serostatus before we first had sex. Eddie feared that I would leave him when he told me he was positive. He felt that his keeping his positive serostatus secret not only was presenting me with a potential health hazard but was also a serious breach of the trust required for any successful relationship. (In some jurisdictions, as mentioned earlier in this book, failure to disclose to a partner that you are HIV positive may also be a violation of the state's criminal law. The failure to disclose your positive status can create civil tort liability as well in the United States and other common law countries.)

Eddie had wanted to tell me earlier, of course, but there never seemed to be a good moment to do that. Until that day he had never told me—and I had never asked. He was healthy and strong and beautiful—a bodybuilder and a former model. Beautiful eyes and a killer smile. I fell into a trap that has ensnared many others: I assumed that if he were positive, he would have volunteered that information before we ever had sex.

To his surprise (and to mine as well, to tell the truth), I told him that his HIV status didn't matter to me. I had many friends with HIV and had had safe sex with many men who were positive or whose status was unknown to me. I was not worried about exposure, because we had been "good boys" and had had only safer sex. I understood that his positive HIV status was a difficult subject for Eddie to bring up and that he was afraid to do it because he was afraid of losing me. (Many HIV-positive persons never disclose their status to their partners because they know that disclosure will often mean the immediate or imminent end of the relationship. There is even anecdotal evidence of HIV-positive teenagers in New York who refuse to use condoms because they believe that using a condom implies the need to do so: use of a condom is an admission of a positive HIV status. To prevent the loss of their love life that would come from disclosing their status, some HIV-positive teenagers thus refuse to use condoms even though they know they are probably infecting their partners.) But while it was difficult for Eddie to tell me his status, it was also difficult for me to ask him about it.

A Prescription for Love

Eddie didn't lose me, despite his disclosure, and we stayed together for about two and a half years. Although relationships end for many reasons, one reason Eddie gave for ending our relationship was that he could no longer deal with being in a positive–negative relationship. He needed to find someone else, and a short time later he did find a wonderful new partner who was also HIV positive. They had seen each other in their doctor's waiting room, and each of them had asked the doctor for the other's name and phone number. Although the doctor would not normally disclose personal information about another patient, the doctor agreed to make an exception this one time because the request had been made by both. The doctor complied by writing out the information on a prescription pad in the examination room—and also providing an apt metaphor for the medical importance of a happy relationship by prescribing a partner on that prescription pad. They lived happily together until Eddie died a few years later.

Reactions and Expectations

My own reaction to Eddie's disclosure of his positive status was not uncommon, but it was probably not typical.

What I think of being "typical" would be Michael's reaction on the TV show *Queer as Folk,* a popular American remake of a successful British TV series. The first year of that series had only one man with HIV, the older, lonely gay brother of Michael's very "proud" mother, who is often shown wearing an "I Love My Gay Son" button to her waitress job. There were no other main characters with HIV during the first year of that program, a strange reality for a show that focuses so intently on the lives of gay men and women who live in a country where many friends and family have HIV. Perhaps the problems and concerns of people living with AIDS do not make for good television, or at least the artificial and carefree environments that the show attempted to create in many of its episodes.

In the second season of the show, the character Michael meets an HIV-positive professor who discloses his status before they have sex. Suprisingly, Michael's normally supportive mother asks her son not to date the professor. Her request that her son not date the man with AIDS is a difficult request for her to make emotionally, in part because she knows that she should not interfere with her son's choice of a partner but also because she is sharing her own home with her brother, who has AIDS. Her request that Michael not date the professor is an implicit rejection of her own brother. In those first episodes, Michael complies with his mother's request and decides to break off the relationship with the man who disclosed that he had HIV. It would seem that HIV brought the end of the relationship before it ever really had a chance to begin. But it was not HIV that ended the relationship: it was pressure from others that ended it.

It was not HIV that ended the relationship: it was the pressure from others.

Like the character Michael, I also had not asked Eddie about HIV. I expected that if he had AIDS that he would just have told me about that. Nothing justified that expectation then. Nothing would justify that expectation now.

But unlike the character Michael in the TV series, I did not end the relationship. I don't know if I would have reacted differently to this news if we were not already two months into our relationship, or if I had not had so many HIV-positive friends, or if I had not participated in as many ACT UP demonstrations in New York as I had. If I had still been living in the sleepy suburbs of Chicago or on the bucolic edge of Lincoln, Nebraska, I probably would have been more afraid when my new partner told me that he had HIV. If I had been a different kind of person, I would have left him the same day I heard the news. (In an earlier relationship when I still lived in Chicago, I was also unfazed when the man I had been dating told me that he had genital herpes. I told him that it was not a problem, given the advances in medications to control the herpes, and that he didn't have to worry about my leaving him. To my disappointment, he left me—and went back to live with his wife.)

A more typical reaction than mine to the disclosure of a positive HIV status may be found in the thoughts expressed by Gordon, a successful Chicago painter and educator who is HIV negative. Gordon is popular in the city and has dated many African American and Latino men. In his comments on whether to date an HIV-positive or HIV-negative man, Gordon said:

"I guess that I just go with the old school and I assume that everyone is positive, so whether somebody is positive or not doesn't really become an issue for me until later on in the relationship.

"When I see that the relationship is going well—when I see that the relationship is going to become more serious—then it does become an issue for me. Up until that point, though, it really isn't an issue [for me] because I'm assuming that he is positive and the kind of sex we'll be having will be more casual. I do think about it, though, when the sex gets more intense.

"Would I go out with an HIV-positive guy? Ideally, I would say yes, that I would, and ideally I really would go out with him. But when it comes right down to it, the answer is a little more gray for me. When you are going to enter into a long-term relationship, you look at things a little closer. Maybe a lot closer.

"But then again HIV isn't the death sentence that it was when I first started dating—how many years ago? People are taking the drugs and they are living longer, and certainly they are outliving most relationships in the gay world anyway.

"So I guess HIV really is an issue for me after all. But if I did find the right guy, I would try to treat him special and to make the relationship important. So, intellectually HIV is probably not an issue for me, but realistically it probably is."

The concluding and conflicting thoughts that Gordon reveals here—that he would probably not want to date an HIV-positive partner—may be found more expressly in the various forums in which people seek out romantic partners. A casual survey of personal advertisements from gay-oriented newspapers, as one example, provides ample evidence of HIV-negative men seeking out only HIV-negative partners:

> NOT YOUR AVERAGE BEAR. We're both independent, introspective, affectionate, expressive, smart [and] successful. Each seeking the other to complement our lives [and] share our values, vision [and] fun. Me: GWM, 45, 5'7", 168#, sexy, hairy, handsome, HIV-neg, bottom. You: 35–55, taller, sensual, hairy, handsome, HIV-neg, top.[3]

> SEEKING GQ WM, HIV-neg, bottom, for possible long-term relationship, 20s to early 30s, who likes rugged hardbody military types, a little rough around the edges, a twist of redneck, very fun, athletic WM, w/brains, very clean cut, not into leather, kink, raunch, or drugs.[4]

> ROMANTIC OPTIMIST. Suburban WM, 49, 6'1", 180#. Laid back, outdoor type, with a sense of humor, but equally comfortable with cultural events. Seeking another HIV-neg WM, 35–55, who is a non-smoker, physically on the thin side [and] may share some of my interests, for possible long-term relationship.[5]

Other advertisements placed by HIV-negative men may stress their health and their interest in long-term romance, factors that would clearly imply to many readers that the HIV-negative man placing the advertisement would not accept an HIV-positive partner. Consider this example:

GWM, 30, HIV-neg, 5'10", 175#, Italian–Irish, ex-gym rat [muscular], sense of humor, likes retro architecture, cars, music, evenings in/out. ISO WM, around 30, relationship-oriented, humorous. No drugs or 17th Street military trendoids please. Some weekdays free a +.[6]

References to HIV do not occur only in personal advertisements but are now also common when meeting others on phone chat lines and in computer bulletin board chat rooms. When HIV is raised as a screen in these contexts, either negatively or positively, its use deepens the viral chasm that divides our community. A man who refuses to meet someone who is HIV positive may be missing out on meeting the partner of his dreams. Yet the many references to HIV status either in personal ads and elsewhere suggest that many people believe that positive should be hooked up to positive and negative to negative, just like jumper cables being attached to car batteries.

The Worried Well: Dreading and Hoping among HIV-Negative Men

These personal advertisements represent a variety of psychological concerns on the part of those who are HIV negative. Many would say that the daily problems faced by people living with HIV are far more important and difficult than the concerns of the worried well. A person who is HIV negative does not generally face daily worries about staying in school, keeping a job, losing health insurance, arranging a complex schedule of drug dosages and doctor visits, losing custody of children, losing a home, and losing friends—all issues that can arise completely aside from the emotional and physical strain of living with HIV.

Yet there are important issues for HIV-negative individuals (and couples), primarily connected to maintaining their seronegative status. HIV is always present psychologically, even when it is absent in reality. As discussed in other chapters in this book, seronegative couples may decide to abandon safer sexual practices in exchange for perceptions of increased intimacy. Discarding safer sexual practices implicates levels of trust that may sometimes be betrayed in a relationship; it is no secret that acts of sexual infidelity have even sometimes reached the White House.

HIV is always present psychologically, even when it is absent in reality.

There are also contributions that HIV-negative individuals (and couples) can make in the fight against AIDS. These contributions go beyond "being a buddy" or raising money at an AIDS Walk or AIDS Ride. For example, sexually active men who remain HIV negative may provide genetic scientists with clues on how to remain uninfected,[7] they may become candidates for vaccine trials, or they may provide AIDS educators and epidemiologists with information on effective educational strategies to prevent the further spread of AIDS. Indeed, providing this information will be crucial as people grow indifferent to safer sex strategies that may have worked in the early years of the pandemic,[8] as sexually awakening teenagers mistakenly perceive HIV as a risk that either affects only an older generation or that has declined in significance because of advances in medicine.[9] Meanwhile conservative cultural or religious norms continue to clash with some of the more explicit public health messages that convey information necessary to help sexually active people protect themselves from AIDS.

A handful of researchers now recognize that there are both psychological needs of persons who are HIV negative and possible benefits in the battle against AIDS from studying the behavior and genetics of HIV-negative men who are sexually active. Two texts, each published in 1995, provide comprehensive studies of issues affecting the uninfected: *In the Shadow of the Epidemic* by Walt Odets[10] and *HIV-Negative: How the Uninfected Are Affected by AIDS* by William I. Johnston.[11]

Survivor's Guilt: Why Am I Still Negative, and Do I Deserve to Be?

"Survivor's guilt" is one of the psychological problems discussed by Odets and Johnston in their books. Odets writes that survivor's guilt is a cornerstone of the psychological problems facing men who are uninfected, and that this guilt plays a central role in the denial of psychological distress among men who are HIV negative.[12] The term *survivor's guilt*, as Johnston explains, first appeared in the literature about survivors of the Nazi Holocaust. The term was later applied to veterans who had returned from the Vietnam War.[13] Johnston finds it natural to apply this term to some HIV-negative men who have difficulty coping with their negative status, because some HIV-negative gay men do not understand why they have avoided the virus when so many other gay men have contracted HIV. Some of these men attribute their HIV-negative status to good luck or to avoiding partners from an older generation that AIDS first devastated. Some men, particularly younger men, may wrongly believe that they have some natural immunity to HIV. Other HIV-negative men who may experience psychological distress at remaining HIV negative may undertake unrelenting commitments to AIDS work as a way of "atoning for their survival, or of punishing themselves for having survived."[14]

> **Sexually active men who remain HIV negative may provide genetic scientists with clues on how to remain uninfected, they may become candidates for vaccine trials, or they may provide AIDS educators and epidemiologists with information on effective educational strategies to prevent the further spread of AIDS.**

Johnston also links survivor's guilt to internalized homophobia and sexual guilt. He writes that when some gay men wonder if they "deserve" to be uninfected, he believes that these men are expressing ambivalence not only about surviving when others have not but also about being gay. Recognizing the rhetoric of some religious leaders who have characterized AIDS as God's punishment, Johnston also notes that some gay men feel unworthy of surviving because they somehow believe that their past (and maybe even their present) sexual behavior deserves to be punished. Johnston writes that during the inexcusable horrors of Nazi Germany and the time of the Holocaust, there were some Jews who could not help feeling that there must be some reason for the unjust persecution that was being inflicted upon them. Johnston believes that in a similar vein, some gay men may also internalize society's persecution of them and imagine that they must somehow "deserve" to contract or suffer from HIV. In this way, Johnston is able to link sexual guilt and internalized homophobia to the guilt that some HIV-negative men may feel as survivors.[15]

Reaching a similar conclusion in his own consideration of internalized homophobia and HIV, Odets writes that for many persons, having AIDS "is much more respectable than being homosexual."[16] Society, the church, and the family can sometimes accept a viral illness more easily than they can accept an alternative sexual orientation. Odets thus observes that "many gay men are finding it easier to be threatened by AIDS, to die of it, or to be guilty for not dying of it, than they have ever found being gay."[17] That observation was likely more true when having a diagnosis of AIDS meant that you didn't have long to live. The thought that it is easier to accept an illness than a sexual orientation may not hold true in a new era when antiretroviral drugs are available to help many people survive for years.

Some gay men feel unworthy of surviving because they somehow believe that their past (and maybe even their present) sexual behavior deserves to be punished.

The act of coming out to family and friends for many individuals will bring questions about their HIV status. Common responses have ranged from "Are you being safe?" to "Do you have AIDS?" Some people will find it easier not to come out than to handle this barrage of questions. Unfortunately, however, when a person cannot "come out" as gay or lesbian, there are likely fewer opportunities to discuss with others feelings of survivor's guilt. Indeed, the inability to help persons with HIV, lest the helper also be branded with a scarlet "AIDS," may actually increase the intensity of survivor's guilt in some individuals.

The survivor's guilt applied by Johnston and Odets to HIV-negative men would also apply to HIV-positive men and women who are long-term survivors. Many HIV-positive persons don't understand why they have outlived so many others, and they question why they respond favorably to protease inhibitor cocktails while the same treatments either fail for others or are unavailable to them.

I don't know why I didn't become infected. I'm lucky, nothing more. I practiced safer sex and learned about HIV and its transmission. Still, there were so many times when I was certain that I was

HIV positive. I will always remember the anxiety of those first few times I went to get an HIV-antibody test. Even though I was well acquainted with how the testing would be done and how long it would take to get the results, I was unprepared for how slowly those days would pass. Waiting for test results was agony, although whatever I may have felt then is of course nothing when compared to the torment I would have faced had those results been positive. I was certain that the results would be positive, and I worked myself into such a frenzy that I even told a friend that I was positive although I had not even received the test results. I felt for lumps that I was sure were there—evidence of slightly enlarged lymph nodes that most likely were just from a sore throat or a cold. I closely examined my tongue and other parts of my body, looking for elusive clues that would disclose evidence of my infection. I felt anxious then; I feel foolish now for that anxiety.

Survivor's guilt and other psychological issues help drive HIV-negative men into the arms of other HIV-negative men. In the company of another with the same seronegative status, a person may not focus on his guilt as an individual survivor but recognize that there are many who have survived. Yet attempts to avoid survivor's guilt are obviously not the only reason that HIV-negative persons seek out HIV-negative partners. Johnston also observed that one of the main reasons that HIV-negative men sought out only other HIV-negative men was that relationships with HIV-positive men "do not seem to offer permanence."[18] He describes one HIV-negative man who said, "I fear the anxiety that I might die as a result of the relationship [with an HIV-positive partner], but I also experience a fear of being left behind, of being left alone. I want to be able to envision myself with my partner ten years from now, even if at any time one of us could be hit by a bus."[19]

Serial Grief: Loss after Loss

Any person who has lost a partner is understandably reluctant to enter into another relationship where it seems likely that the new partner will also die. This concept of "serial grief" is serious enough when applied to friend after friend who is lost to AIDS; when the person lost was a life partner, the serial grief can be unbearable. The problem of serial loss is often ignored by those outside the gay community or other communities that are heavily hit by infection with HIV.[20] Consider, for example, another personal advertisement from a gay newspaper in Washington, DC:

> LOOKING FOR LOVE. Professional WM, 47, 175#, 6', HIV-negative, thinning light brown hair and mustache. Lost lover of 9 years (4 years ago) and am ready to get on with life. Decent, friendly, caring and somewhat shy (raised in a small New England town). Looking for relationship. Love intimate times, quiet walks, weekend getaways and city life (sidewalk cafes, theater, museums, dancing, etc.). Dislikes are bar groupies, born-agains, and smokers.[21]

In speculating about the person behind the advertisement, gay readers would assume that the man placing the ad had lost his partner to AIDS. This assumption may or may not be correct; it will be an assumption made nonetheless in the context of this ad and the newspaper in which it was placed. Including the information about a lover lost four years ago was not strictly necessary for the ad, for it would have functioned equally well without that sentence. If the man were straight and heterosexually married, he could have written "widower." Persons in same-sex relationships often do not have the verbal luxury of words to convey the true scope of their relationships.

The problem of serial loss is often ignored by those outside the gay community or other communities that are heavily hit by infection with HIV.

Although the man does not limit responses to those who are HIV negative, he includes his own HIV status in addition to the information about his lost lover. The combination of words would imply to many readers that this man is not seeking a relationship with an HIV-positive man. Yet, having gone this far in the analysis, close readers may also assume that the man would not necessarily reject a response from a potential partner who was positive if the respondent's other attributes were sufficiently intriguing. He had a lover of nine years and presumably had been through the normal ups and downs of a relationship, whatever they may be. Indeed, the man has not specified any requirements for his potential partner other than his desire to avoid drunks, smokers, and born-again fundamentalist Christians. Some may say that the lack of express requirements reflects his openness to love in whatever form it may come. If he were to find an HIV-negative partner, however, it would be reasonable to assume that the advertiser, who had been in a nine-year relationship, would expect a certain level of commitment from his new partner.

When an HIV-negative person hooks up with another HIV-negative person, there is often an expectation of mutual fidelity and monogamy. Johnston notes that many couples "are not sexually exclusive, so some men in negative–negative couples practice protected sex because they are not certain that their outside sexual contacts are safe. For such men, insisting on practicing safer sex within the couple is a sign of their commitment to each other's health."[22]

A Practical Trust:
Staying Together and Staying Safe

Men may stray. But negative guys want to stay negative and not infect their partners if they do go astray. So many negative–negative couples practice safer sex. In addition to mutual respect for each other's health, Johnston identifies "personal control" as one reason that an HIV-negative man gave for insisting on safer sex with his negative partner.[23] He didn't want to trust another person with his life by having unprotected sex. Remaining within his own guidelines for safer sex, the man believed he would keep control over his own HIV status. He recognized that insisting on having only safer sex with his partner could be interpreted as being unable to commit to him fully, but for this man—and many others—it was infinitely more important to keep absolute control over his own HIV status.[24] Johnston concludes that this man's comment reflects "an important truth about relationships in the time of AIDS: Without trust, unprotected sex with an HIV-negative partner feels dangerous."[25]

This danger of unprotected sex is undeniably attractive to some. *Barebacking,* discussed in Chapter 4, is often common in negative–negative relationships. According to the theoretical justifications for barebacking in a negative–negative relationship, if both partners are negative then there can be no risk of HIV transmission.

The problem with this theory is that we do not always know that both partners are *truly negative.* First, there is a window period during which a person exposed to the HIV antigen will not yet have developed the HIV antibodies tested for in standard ELISA (enzyme-linked immunosorbent assay) and Western Blot tests. An infected person may seroconvert after the blood is drawn. Second, despite protestations to the contrary about the accuracy of the test, there are human factors of error and biological reasons that still sometimes produce false-negative test results. Third, and most important, while a person who tests negative will know that his individual behavior has maintained that HIV-negative status, he cannot know that for his sexual partner. Monogamy may be promised but is never guaranteed. For these reasons, the presumed safety of barebacking is a false presumption. To put it bluntly, barebacking is fucking stupid! Too many have died and too many have been infected to ignore the obvious lesson: *if it is within our power to preserve our own health and the health of those we love, we have to play it safe.*

Yet for long-term couples who are convinced of their unwavering monogamy, questions of supposedly increased intimacy and implied trust come up against the position presented here—that it is better to be safe than sorry. The Australian sexologist and author Dennis Altman of La Trobe University (Melbourne) has argued that in many gay relationships a promise of monogamy is nothing but a false promise. He believes that "gay relationships are not based upon an assumption of monogamy"[26] and that even in the age of AIDS "monogamy is not a realistic choice for many of us."[27]

While strict monogamy is obviously the ideal in public health terms for an HIV-negative couple, there is still the threat that one of the partners may slip up at some point and place both at risk. As the Clinton White House scandal demonstrated, it is not always easy to admit to an "inappropriate relationship" outside of marriage. Because there is always a chance that a partner may stray or that monogamy may be defined or understood differently in different relationships (see Chapter 6), there is still a chance of infection with HIV. For this reason, as Johnston observes, "HIV has so infiltrated the consciousness of gay men that it has a virtual presence even in the lives of the uninfected."[28]

Of course, there are and will continue to be many couples who commit to exclusive relationships and who keep those vows (see the box). The litigation in Hawaii and the legislation in Vermont have even gotten us used to the idea of committed relationships sanctioned by law. The specter of AIDS can even help keep the relation-

NEGOTIATED SAFETY: TALK, TEST, TEST, TALK

The practice in which two HIV-negative partners decide to forgo condoms and agree to either monogamy or engaging only in specific safer behaviors with others outside the relationship has been called "negotiated safety." One model recently developed in Australia for such a practice is "Talk, Test, Test, Talk." The model with two tests in the middle factors in the time lag that occurs between exposure, conversion, and the body developing antibodies that will be picked up on an HIV test. "Talk" is key in determining what new sexual behaviors (or perhaps return to older ones) the couple will engage in. It also leaves the door open to communicate if, after the negative test result, a slipup occurs within the relationship or there is potential risk to reliability of their negative status (e.g., sex with someone outside the relationship and a condom break occurs). The couple, for example, may resume condom usage and begin the cycle of testing again to help insure that their negative status will be maintained. The Australian model is a response to the reality that many fall off the safer-sex wagon. It is also a reaction to the fear that a person who must go through his whole sexual life with condoms eventually feels this is a task that seems too daunting; such a fatalistic expectation often translates into unplanned and unprotected sex.

ship monogamous by making it too risky to stray too far from the home port. This view of potentially increased rates of monogamy found early support in predictions made by David P. McWhirter and Andrew M. Mattison, the authors of *The Male Couple*. They found that although there was evidence "indicating lack of sexual exclusivity among male couples, we believe that there is a trend toward more sexual exclusivity in the future."[29] They predicted that fear of AIDS would propel a trend toward monogamy, and noted also that "there is a more conservative undercurrent flowing, and more and more individuals are expressing the desire for sexual exclusivity with just one other man."[30] Their writings seem to have anticipated not only the later writings of socially conservative theorists such as Bruce Bawer and Andrew Sullivan but also many aspects of the public debate that would arise in the wake of the first same-sex marriage decision from the Hawaii Supreme Court, which ruled that the refusal to grant marriage licenses to same-sex couples in Hawaii violated the the Hawaii State Constitution before it was amended.[31]

Public Health and Economic Arguments
for Same-Sex Marriage

In addition to the predictions of increased monogamy made by
McWhirter and Mattison in *The Male Couple,* there have been legal
and even economic arguments raised to support stable monogamous relationships as a public health measure. One example of a legal argument to support the legality of same-sex relationships is
found in an article by Michael L. Closen and Carol R. Heise, who argued that the state should permit gay marriages as a public health
measure to reduce the spread of HIV.[32] They argued that when couples could enjoy the legal stability of a recognized marriage, there
would be less risk of spreading HIV. Closen and Heise's argument
assumes that those same-sex marriages would be monogamous and
furthermore that each of the partners in those marriages would be
HIV negative. Those assumptions will not always be true.

Other arguments for same-sex marriage were made in addition
to the public health argument. As an example of an economic argument that also supports the concept of same-sex marriage, econo-
mist Tomas J. Philipson and Judge Richard A. Posner of the U.S.
Court of Appeals for the Seventh Circuit observed that "fear of contracting AIDS induces people to substitute marital for nonmar-
ital sex because the former is safer."[33] Because allowing gay marriages would increase monogamy and decrease the spread of HIV,
Philipson and Posner argue, "states should authorize homosexual
marriage in order to reduce the cost of [a form of] safe sex."[34] Continuing further with their assumptions of negative–negative relationships free of marital infidelity, they argue that restructuring the
federal tax code would help reduce the spread of AIDS. Philipson
and Posner argue that "subsidizing marriage through generous tax
exemptions for married people would reduce the spread of AIDS
by reducing the amount of promiscuous sex."[35] Reflecting an im-
probable intersection of sexual orientation and the federal tax
code, however, they also argue that the "marriage [tax] subsidy"
must be given equally to heterosexuals and homosexuals because to
give it only to heterosexually married couples would supposedly "in-
duce male homosexuals to marry women at an even greater rate
than they do, and bisexual activity is an important source of transmission of the AIDS virus to women."[36] I do *not* care what kind of
tax break Philipson and Posner are willing to give me; it will not be

enough for me to change my sexual orientation. It is interesting to note that they make no assumption of monogamy for gay men who would marry women for the supposed tax advantages, although they do make this assumption for partners in a same-sex marriage.

We have considered the legal and economic arguments raised to support same-sex marriage as a tool of public health to reduce the further spread of AIDS. To be fair, neither Closen and Heise nor Philipson and Posner would argue that their positions infinitely guarantee the fidelity or negative serostatus of partners in a state-authorized marriage. Additionally, many HIV-negative persons recognize that they still may become HIV-positive at any time. Their negative HIV status may be nothing more than a temporary status that can vanish at any moment.

Because there is no guarantee of a continuing negative viral status, some persons will react by taking extra care to preserve their negative status. Others will take risks, such as barebacking, because they may see that their negative status can change at any time. The division is similar to the future marriages of children whose parents divorce: for some children, their later marriage will not work out because their parents' marriage did not work out; for other children, their later marriage *will* work out because they feel that they have to do a better job than their parents did. The same phenomenon is seen with children of alcoholics: some become alcoholics because their parents were alcoholics, whereas others would never touch a drink because they saw how alcohol destroyed their parents. Just as with responses to HIV, the psychological reactions can be completely different in different persons.

Although the work of Odets and Johnston provided the groundwork for understanding many of the problems faced by HIV-negative persons in the age of AIDS, their work has not produced large-scale responses to this population group. As Eric Rofes observes in *Dry Bones Breathe: Gay Men Creating Post-AIDS Identities and Cultures*, although the books by Odets and Johnston "were both well-received and reviewed, they do not appear to have initiated long-term qualitative studies aimed at understanding the continuing challenges faced by HIV-negative gay men as they attempt to make meaning of the epidemic."[37] Perhaps the reason for this lies with the disease itself, as drug companies do not want to fund studies of HIV-negative men, who won't be spending money on AIDS drugs.

FIVE WAYS TO ASK

The number of partners a person has had is an indication only of promiscuity, not of HIV status. A person who has had sex only once before may be HIV positive. What matters more now is what the person's status is. Here are some ways to ask about HIV status:

1. Are you negative or positive? When were you tested?
2. If you were positive, would you tell me?
3. I'm negative. Are you?
4. Are you safe? (Good, let's keep it that way.)
5. The answer won't change how I feel about you, but I need to know. Are you HIV-positive?

While those studies may still be yet to come, the HIV-negative persons who "live in the shadow of AIDS" will continue to do so whether or not they are formally studied. As this chapter has noted, many of them will do so in the company of other HIV-negative men (see the box). Yet, as Johnston concludes, "One of the greatest challenges facing HIV-negative gay men these days is to find a way to celebrate their futures and build lives worth living, without feeling that by doing so they are abandoning the HIV-positive. To embrace life is not to dishonor those who have died or give affront to those who are ill."[38] Although I am HIV negative, I am a person living with AIDS because I live in a society that is living with AIDS. I will not abandon my friends or my community, even though I may find happiness in the arms of a partner who also happens to be HIV negative. We didn't ask each other about our viral status when we first met—that was only a secondary factor after the primary question of love.

SIX

IN SICKNESS AND IN HEALTH
Your Body and Your Relationship

There comes a time in a couple's life together when they can go either of two ways: stay together or break up. Each way is equally valid. When I work with a couple, it's important to know if their goal is to strengthen the relationship or to terminate it with grace. Asking this for yourself and as a couple will crystallize for you what kind of work you want to do in your relationship.

Too often couples in a crisis, whether triggered by HIV or something else, end up immobilized in an unsatisfactory relationship based on obligation instead of commitment because they are unable to communicate and solve problems. I've seen this happen over and over, despite the love that both partners profess for each other.

Love, it turns out, does not conquer all.

Veterans of long-term relationships already know this. But many of us do not, especially if our relationships have been relatively brief in the past, and now, with the harbinger that is HIV, we've become interested in long-term commitment for the first time. If you're an incurable romantic, you may believe that undying love is all you and your partner need to stay together and happy, now that you've found each other. But as a former colleague of mine, Johanne Arsenequilt, LCSW, of Pride Institute, tells her patients, "Love is not enough; you also need the ability to communicate and problem-solve."

In this chapter several diverse couples explain how they have stayed together through physical illness, how they have weathered relationship crises as individuals, and how their romantic lives have evolved over the years.

As you're reading this book, you may already subscribe to the idea that being in a relationship that works or can be repaired is desirable for a wide variety of reasons. One of those reasons may very well be the health benefits that I've mentioned earlier. If so, keep in mind that when we talk about the healing power of love, we mean love in a healthy, affirming relationship. A stressful, abusive, or otherwise unhealthy relationship is likely to counteract the health benefits of whatever love has existed between two people.

The Healing Power of Love in a Healthy Relationship

Early in our relationship my former partner, Jerry, went to his doctor to have his T-cell count done. "Well, it went up 33 percent, from 8 to 11, since I met you," he smiled while reporting his lab work. If a nurturing relationship confers health on the partners, then the converse is also true. I recall the changes in my T-cell and viral load count after Jerry's death. In February 1997, before the frequent trips to the hospital and acceleration of his disease, my T-cell count was 380 with a viral load of 21,000. In October, two months after his death, my T-cell count was 108 with a viral load that had skyrocketed to 604,000. My physician said this was not unusual after the stress of being a caregiver and the subsequent reaction to loss (she was also Jerry's physician and present along with me and his family when he died).

Understanding this to be true, I wonder if my health would have suffered to that degree if we had only broken up—if my health would have declined as much because I had lost a personal confidant, no matter the cause.

HIV has given us a good opportunity to witness the healing power of love informally, but now the conventional wisdom that an affirming relationship contributes both longevity and well-being to those involved is being supported by science. Cardiologist and author Dean Ornish, in his book *Love and Survival: The Scientific Basis for the Healing Power of Intimacy*, states, "Our survival depends on the healing power of love, intimacy and relationships."[1] Isolation and lack of purpose and meaning is as great a predictor of illness and mortality as a bout with pneumonia. Being cut off from others may perhaps protect us from their sneezes, but in that isolation we increase the risk for other more devastating ills.

Ornish cites more than a hundred medical studies that link our relationships with our health. Asking the question "Does your wife show you her love?" researchers from Case Western Reserve University studied 10,000 men to see who would develop angina pectoris (chest pains triggered by a heart disorder) over a five-year period (men selected were deemed at high risk due to family history, high cholesterol count, etc.). Those who answered yes were less than half as likely to develop chest pains as those who answered no. At Duke University, doctors studied the survival rate of 1,400 men and women who were found to have at least one severely blocked artery. Five years later, 50 percent of those who had been unmarried and had stated they had no one they could talk to on a regular basis about their lives were dead. Only 15 percent of those who had been married or had a confidant died in the same time period. Similar connections between health and intimacy have been found for illnesses that range from ulcers to cancer.

After Jerry died, my numbers improved owing to the encouragement of family and friends and my going on the protease cocktail. This experience gave me a greater understanding of the mutual healing that can occur in a strong relationship. The amount of support present in a relationship is something I try to assess while working with my positive patients who come to therapy as couples. I also look at the amount of validation a couple receives from outside the relationship—be it from workmates, friends, or family—in assessing the future health of the relationship and the people in it.

A Vaccinated Lover

At no other time has science so intersected our lives—or, more precisely, our love lives.

I met Dirk, a botanist, while sailing on the Potomac on a Saturday in August. We were both members of a gay and lesbian sailing group. As he struggled to captain our small boat in the absence of wind, we eventually discussed the book I was working on. Several months later he told me that the new love in his life happened to be HIV positive and he had decided to involve himself in an additional kind of medical safety net. "I did it partly out of curiosity—as there are a lot of medical people in my family," Dirk said. His decision was based mainly, of course, on his own realization of increased risk now that he had an HIV-positive boyfriend.

> If you are interested in more information about becoming a volunteer in a HIV vaccine study, check out the website *www.hvtn.org* or call the AIDS Clinical Trials Information Service at 1-800-TRIALSA.

The decision was to enroll in an HIV vaccine trial (see the box): "Up till now I have tested negative, and though we practice safe sex, we both wanted to keep me negative."

In this chapter we discuss the importance of care for yourself and the mutuality of care between you and your partner. My work has shown that seroconversion or infection of a partner is an obstacle that some couples cannot overcome. An effective vaccine or broader barrier choices, including virucidal creams or foams, would help to maintain the health and length of the relationship. It could also increase people's willingness to partner with us without having to worry about their own health risks.

Long-Term Survivors . . . of Relationships

> *When I was a boy I would collect leaves and press them in heavy books like dictionaries and Bibles. Spending the day in a park with a friend of mine I noticed some bright red leaves that I wanted to press between those pages. Those leaves were wrapped around an oak tree. He said, "Don't touch those, it's poison ivy."*
>
> —Unknown

Bright red was also the color of the living room walls in this couple's DC row house. They had been together for fourteen years, and in the fifteenth year of their relationship they found out they are both HIV positive.

Sal is a fifty-year-old marine engineer who was raised in Rhode Island. He has the build of a comfortable married man and the satisfaction of knowing he is in the kind of relationship that many men with more defined physiques hope one day to have. He is more outgoing and eager to talk than his partner, Kirk. Kirk is forty-two, slimmer and fairer in complexion than Sal, is from West Virginia, and works in marketing.

"We met in a bar on a Friday night, and we moved in together on Sunday," recalls Sal. "I was also a little high that night."

"I remember Sal telling me, 'If it wasn't so hot in here, I would ask you to a dance,' and he bought me a drink instead," Kirk told us.

When I expressed some surprise at the rapid sequence of events, Sal replied, "I just went home to get my car and moved in from there. I hardly thought about it."

"Oz was the name of that bar outside Fort Bragg," Kirk remembers as his eyes look upward, seeking additional memories. He then adds quickly, "We were both in the Army at the time. It was March 1984. AIDS was unknown then, at least to the Army, and Fort Bragg is an Army town, so if the Army didn't know about it, we didn't either."

"My XO [executive officer] knew about Kirk," Sal said. He then pointed to the windows that encircle the crimson turret of his living room. "Yeah . . . he even made the blinds for us, and he is straight and very accepting of our relationship."

"I was a paramedic, and even I knew there was not even a program or test yet in the military," Kirk emphasized.

I asked if they had been discharged from the military because of their HIV status. Sal replied, "I was tested while I served in the Reserves. They were doing random testing then, so I thought I'd get the jump on them and went to my doctor in 1988. . . . I was still negative in '88." A decade later that was no longer the case.

Unlike Sal, Kirk waited quite a while before he was tested: "I was never tested until a year ago. When I broke out in hives that covered my entire body, my doctor suggested a test. It cleared up while I awaited the results, but then it returned on my leg—I panicked."

Sal quietly offers, "We found out within a week . . . that I was too."

I asked them the first thought that came to my mind: "Were you monogamous in your relationship?" Kirk responded, "We had seen people in open relationships and saw it not working. . . . We both saw what it did."

Sal continued, "We also never used condoms." That last statement prompted me to recall the HIV prevention messages early in the pandemic that encouraged monogamy. The problem was that the ads often failed to clarify that both partners must be negative for monogamy to be fully effective in preventing HIV. Sal believes that Kirk was the one who gave him HIV, based on the following: "My T-cells after the test were five hundred, Kirk's were one hundred," he said. Kirk elaborated as to his own cause of infection: "I spent six months stationed in New Jersey in 1982 when that mysterious disease was raging across the country, traveling from person to person." He also recalled that "the baths were popular then, as they are again."

When asked about the changes in their relationship since their diagnoses, Kirk offered, "Your emotions are overwhelmed. . . . You begin to imagine the worst-case scenarios." While coming to realize his health status was now fragile, he said, "Everyone is walking around with something, either a disease or some toxin, and we can't do much about it. Facing your mortality helps you know your place in life."

This statement about lack of control contrasts with the couple's attempts to live—at least when they were first diagnosed—a healthier life. "For me it was an awakening. I gave up smoking, began going to the gym, and started eating fat-free potato chips," said Sal. Kirk joins in: "We lost a taste for alcohol as a result of the medicine. But luckily it came back," he added, exaggerating the clinking of ice cubes in his cocktail.

The initial rush to health is very common postdiagnosis, and people are able to maintain it to varying degrees. I still have dusty bottles of papaya enzyme, Chinese herbs, and a half bottle of vitamin E in a box somewhere; I have no recollection what papaya enzyme is good for, but I'm surviving without it.

In discussing their sex lives Sal explains, "We have always been open and communicative about sex, and we didn't cheat. The advent of computer online services caused us to consider having brief three-way relationships, and we had five of them from April until December in 1998, when we found out. Any change in our sexual behaviors has been due to the computer, not HIV."

Kirk pipes up, "We played safe with those people."

Sal continues, "We resumed this again, but only with positive people. . . . I don't think, uh, I could have sex with an uninfected person." These last statements clearly are in conflict with what the couple said earlier about being strictly monogamous—having sex only with each other.

The Rules: Explicit or Implicit

However, what is clear is that both men have come to an understanding that is based on a bedrock of emotional fidelity, while also allowing a sexual fluidity within their relationship. This openness is something that many gay men are able to achieve either through communication and outlining rules and expectations or by trial and error. The risk with the latter, of course, is that if you have unstated beliefs or very contrasting expectations, they get put to the test when one of you gets caught literally "with your pants down."

> *In a society where we cannot marry, by definition* all *of our relationships are extra-marital.*
> —David Nimmons, *The Soul Beneath the Skin*

Kirk and Sal have chosen expanded monogamy. By defining what works for them (namely, to have three-way sex encounters with other HIV-positive men) they exercise a commitment to the relationship, while also working within their own value system of not spreading HIV further into the community. While certainly HIV has caused many gay men to reconsider the whole question of monogamy, according to one study approximately two-thirds of gay men were indeed still in open relationships.[3]

When asked about the additional rules in their relationship, Kirk stated, "A no violence rule. . . . I grew up with parents arguing. Yell all you want; it gets it out."

When asked about their relationships with their families and their families' support of their relationship, Kirk continued, "My family didn't like Sal, and my mother was convinced he'd converted me to homosexuality. I had to tell her about our relationship

According to one study approximately two-thirds of gay men were still in open relationships.

FROM OPEN TO EXCLUSIVE: VARIATIONS OF MONOGAMY

Here are some variations of monogamy for gay men defined by G. D. Travers Scott in his essay "Flexible Fidelity," contained in the anthology *Gay Men at the Millennium*[2]—

- *Rose-Colored Monogamy:* No sexual or romantic contact with anyone outside the relationship.
- *Pragmatic Monogamy:* Sexual exclusivity but tolerance for social kissing, affection, and flirtation, as well as open acknowledgment of desire. You can dish and rubberneck together, but not act on those desires.
- *Virtual Monogamy:* No physical sex outside [the] relationship, but porn, Internet, videos, phone sex, etc., are OK.
- *Expanded Monogamy:* Sexual exclusivity except for bringing home mutually agreed-upon and shared third parties.
- *Sleazy Monogamy:* No hardcore sex outside of the relationship, only quick, anonymous, public jerk-offs to vent steam.
- *Out of Sight, Out of Mind:* Having sex outside the relationship only when separated by distance.
- *Variation: Don't Ask, Don't Tell:* You may not want to tell each other about your separate activities until reunited, in order to avoid getting competitive and trying to outdo one another.
- *Open, with Exceptions*: Full-fledged sex with others is OK, but you and your partner negotiate limits of intimacy to be respected. You might want strict top/bottom arrangements with outside partners or no experimenting with activities not already established in your sexual repertoire.
- *Open but Anonymous:* Everything up to and including full-fledged hardcore sex is OK, allowing for [bathhouses] and tricking, but only with strangers: no friends, no exes, no repeats, nothing prearranged.
- *Boomerang:* Do whatever you want, but always come home.
- *Anything Goes:* Complete and unrestrained whoredom.

so Mom could get to know Sal." Sal elaborated, "You told her during your aunt's funeral." Kirk smiled. "That was bad timing." Kirk continued, "I've never told my father, who was also a career soldier, but now Sal and Dad e-mail each other, so it works out smoothly. Neither of my parents knows about our HIV status."

Sal said, "My mother found out about his HIV status the day I did. She hasn't changed, except every three months she asks, 'What

are the numbers?' and every time CNN does a TV segment on
AIDS she summarizes it for me."

I smiled and recalled a conversation with my own mother
whom I told four years after I found out that I was HIV positive and
the same week my partner died. She now says, "Mikey, I saw on the
news today about a new AIDS drug treatment." When I inquire as
to the name of the treatment, she replies in a Southern drawl, "I
didn't catch that, honey, but I'm sure your doctor knows about it."
Then she asks me what my numbers are, as she is usually convinced
I am shielding her from bad news.

On reflection, this couple who had been together in a solid relationship for fourteen years had found out something that might
have torn apart or fiercely united a different couple with less shared
history. With this bedrock of commitment, they did not have to face
some of the same fears and possible stigmatization as would those
who are single or just beginning a relationship. This couple can survive the "autumn" of their relationship, which includes HIV, and
continue to enjoy rolling in the crimson leaves together.

Untaken Vows: Commitment without Recognition

Gay men living with HIV have a lot of obstacles to deal with in trying to maintain a healthy relationship while also maintaining their
own physical health. A big one is the fact that we usually cannot
marry. How can we hope to have affirming relationships when society refuses to affirm our commitment to each other?

The *Advocate*, in a June 1998 article about monogamy, stated,
"The fact remains that society celebrates heterosexual monogamy
with legal weddings, newspaper announcements, and unquestion-
ing joy, while gay marriage is so controversial that its very existence
must be decided by the courts."[4] (Note: *The New York Times* began
running commitment ceremony announcements in 2002, signaling
a trend that I hope many other newspapers will follow.) Ray and
Andy have the appearance of being married, but not the legal sanc-
tion and benefits. This adds stress to already stressful lives and
threatens the health of the relationship that is helping each maxi-
mize his own physical health.

In 1991, three Hawaiian couples, two lesbian and one gay, sued
after their marriage licenses were denied by the state. Two years

later, the Hawaiian Supreme Court ruled—in *Baehr v. Lewin*—that these couples could be legally married under that state's current constitution. The high court also said that the couples' right to marriage was based on gender discrimination rules, not sexual discrimination rules. In the November 1998 elections, voters in Hawaii turned out in big numbers and 58 percent cast ballots supporting the antigay initiative designed to give the state legislature the power and the go-ahead to change the state constitution to limit legal recognition of marriage to heterosexual couples. Alaskans also voted to amend their state constitution to ban legal recognition of gay marriages. That same November, South Carolina removed a 103-year-old law that banned interracial marriages. The now moot law was testament to the tenacity of this type of discrimination.

After Hawaii recognized in its Supreme Court ruling the state's discrimination and bias in favor of male–female couples, many other state legislatures, in response, have enacted laws to prevent gay marriages from occurring.

For couples who literally have to deal with the "in sickness and health" part of wedding vows, this inability to marry has numerous negative implications. Access to spousal benefits are denied, such as health insurance, the Family Medical Leave Act (note: some states, including the District of Columbia, do recognize the rights of domestic partners to medical leave—consult with a local attorney), bereavement leave, and inheritance rights. For gay/lesbian couples extra legal steps need to be taken to acquire, preserve, or attempt to duplicate these benefits. A fuller discussion of these issues is included in Appendix A by legal expert Liz Seaton.

Money Issues:
Even More Stressful for Gay Couples

It's often said that money and sex are the two biggest stressors and causes for arguments in a relationship. This is doubly true for gay couples. First, legal rights to survivorship and other benefits of marriage are often denied to gay couples, making their financial dealings more complicated than for heterosexual spouses. But, secondly, HIV often has a negative financial impact on the positive individual's life and, by extension, on the couple and family (see the box). The disparity in health status alone can cause or exagger-

THE COST OF AIDS

Each HIV infection costs society $154,000 in lifetime treatment costs. Add the impact of Social Security, disability, and insurance payments, and you're up to a quarter of a million dollar for individual infections.

Ninety-four percent of the world's population with HIV does not have access to expensive new drug treatments, according to findings presented at the Fourteenth International Conference on AIDS held in Barcelona, Spain, in July 2002. Even if HIV could be treated with just a clean, clear glass of water, millions of people living with HIV in many parts of the world would not be able to access it.

ate inequity in the partners' earning power and financial stability, which seems to contribute to underlying tension between them, as the couples introduced later in this chapter demonstrate.

As a social worker I often encourage my clients to see that the economic devastation that this disease will create cannot be underestimated and to plan accordingly.

On the flip side, for others, HIV can offer new and different financial opportunities. Many gay magazines and newspapers are flooded with Viatical company ads. Viatical comes from the Latin word "viaticum," which is an allowance for traveling or final expenses. This relatively new industry revolves around the sale of or cashing out of life insurance policies, where someone with a terminal illness is given a percentage of the face value of the policy based on a projected life expectancy, history of illness, etc. However, it should be noted that now that new treatments are available the percentage paid on these policies has gone down dramatically except for the most seriously ill.

A colleague of mine, Gloria Grening Wolk, MSW, who has helped me through the sale of my policy, writes about the benefits and pitfalls of these transactions in her book *Cash for the Final Days.*[5] This financial guide for the terminally ill is a valuable resource to accessing a unique and reliable financial resource.

The Financial Benefit of Knowing Your Status

One of the benefits of testing and knowing your HIV status is to begin to plan for a time when either you are not working or will need financial assistance. I know after my own diagnosis I became more conscious of saving and investing, considering what kind of benefits my employers and government could offer, and realizing that relying on just one stream of income was not sufficient.

A good social worker can help navigate many of these questions—whether it is qualifying for Social Security disability payments, AIDS Drug Assistance programs, or rental assistance.

Additional avenues for help include organizations that can supply you with home-delivered meals. There are even groups that help with dog food. One such group, PETS DC, is where I adopted one of my two dogs, Georgia, a sad-eyed, protective beagle mix whose human mother had died of AIDS. Georgia is particularly vicious toward anything that comes through my mail slot, and I have sent many a bill payment out with teeth marks that I try to assure the utility companies are not mine.

Tips from Your CPA: Certified Positive Accountant

- *The emergency fund.* Look at your current savings. If you or your partner suddenly became ill, would you have enough money to tide you over for six months? Though you may not have been a strong saver in the past, the need to plan for that contingency is vital if you are positive.
- *Retirement planning.* As gay men, whether positive or not, we have to approach investing a little differently than our straight and/or healthy friends. It is likely that many of us will not have children to assist in our care and other needs. For those of us in relationships, the lack of survivorship benefits in noncontributory employer pensions and Social Security has to be taken into account when doing that planning. This means we may need to invest more money than other folks and potentially have less time to accumulate those funds in our IRAs and 401k plans. The time to start is now, I even got into the habit of increasing my 401k deferments whenever I got less than stellar lab reports. My motto is "when T-cells go down—savings go up."
- *Disability insurance.* See if your employer provides this, or when switching jobs look at this as an especially attractive benefit when deciding among potential job offers. Also, if you are considering retiring soon due to health, enroll or activate disability insurance on your credit cards and loans. By

doing this last piece of planning one couple I counseled were able to wipe out legally $80,000 in loans using "credit disability insurance."

- *Legal matters.* The court system, health care system, and financial service providers often adhere to a traditional definition of family that may not recognize your relationship. Hence, you will need to create the necessary legal documents, from simply opening a joint checking account that allows your partner to continue paying the bills to keeping the money flowing in via direct deposit for Social Security if you are retired. (Note: Powers of attorney can authorize another to do the same if you are single.) That way you make sure everything is taken care of, from paying the mortgage to keeping the lights turned on. Also see Appendix A for a more in-depth coverage of this subject, including wills and estate planning.
- *Introduce him to the folks.* Whether it means coming out as gay and letting your family and straight friends/coworkers know this or sharing your HIV status, letting others know how important he is to you and your health and well-being will make them more likely to respect your input and treat him as a full and equal partner.

If you plan wisely, you can minimize the financial impact this disease can have and maybe take your sweetie on that dream honeymoon you both deserve.

Can Illness Strengthen a Relationship?

We've already met couples in earlier chapters who were wrestling with how a disparity in health status would shift the balance of power and force a redefinition of their roles, making them look at their feelings about giving and receiving care. Juan and Angel have stayed together for 25 years—first as lovers and now as friends and roommates. HIV (acting as a type of emotional glue) has kept them together. They admit that they would not be living together if it wasn't for Juan's severe illness.

Juan and Angel are making an attempt to move apart from the lover aspect of their relationship. Though they still live together and Angel is definitely Juan's primary caregiver, Angel has been involved with another man for four years and Juan has begun dating.

We went to visit them in their townhouse, which Angel owns, cloistered away in a complex in the heart of the city. They've lived there for quite a while. It is a lived-in home with two yapping dogs they call their "children." We were escorted to the small dining room, and while I set up my computer, they hunched at the opposite end of the table and began to share their story.

Though Juan is older than Angel and is still weak from "wasting syndrome" from which he almost died three years ago, and is now unemployed and financially dependent on Angel, he didn't seem to feel any shame or inferiority about this.

What they have preserved is still a marriage of sorts.

"When I became sick, Angel became my caregiver, my everything. He supported me financially, emotionally, even though Angel was having sex outside the relationship," Juan told us. "Illness has strengthened our relationship."

Latin Lovers: Shared Culture and Serostatus

In fact, they have a lot in common. Both are positive. Both are Latino. Both have traveled outside the country to meet each other's family: Angel is from Ecuador; Juan is from Chile. They are of similar culture and mind. They even prefer the same toothpaste and soap.

"There is a cultural connection, an educational connection between Angel and me," Juan said. Angel has a PhD in zoology; Juan has one in Spanish literature.

"Angel is my first and only Latino lover. I talk to him in Spanish. We are more like siblings, like family."

"He is like my uncle or brother," Angel added. "Juan and I never broke up mentally. We have separate bedrooms. But I feel more committed to Juan than to Kevin [his new lover]. I would drop Kevin for Juan."

But in the next breath, Angel says that Juan just met someone and had started to date him, and Angel "likes that."

The role that Angel plays for Juan extends even to health care decisions. Angel has power of health care attorney for Juan. No one has power of health care attorney for Angel, though Angel's new lover is the executor of his will: "Juan is not in a stable situation to take care of things. He's not capable emotionally. Kevin is more savvy; he is an investment adviser."

Where some might label their relationship as codependent—including their gay American friends who tell Angel that Juan is a "leech" and advise him to break away—Angel and Juan themselves describe their relationship as one of nurturance.

Juan has retired, has become "a housewife, shops, does the errands, not enough of the dishes," according to Angel, "and some of the cooking." The house is Angel's: he makes the payments; he says he works all day and does more than his share of the housework, "but I would never throw him out," he explained. "I see myself as living with Juan for the rest of my life. I don't know if I'm capable of moving away."

In many Latino cultures, it is not uncommon to keep a mistress. Their shared culture affords Angel and Juan a degree of tolerance that others may not have.But this unusual commitment is not without its strains. Angel is on a tight schedule of how he divides his time between Juan and Kevin. Number one rule: Kevin never spends the night at Angel and Juan's house, even though Juan says, "It wouldn't bother me if he did," though he doesn't talk too favorably of Kevin. "We tolerate each other," Juan admits.

Angel spends Friday and Saturday nights and Sunday days with Kevin. But he comes back every morning to check on Juan and walk the dogs.

Though the last time they shared a bed together was in 1993, Angel and Juan still spend every Christmas and Thanksgiving together.

"Juan is my lover without the sex," Angel explained. "I have two lovers, two lives. Kevin is more of my part-time lover," he qualified after thinking it over. But the confusion persists. Angel wears a ring from Kevin. After all, they have been together for four years.

How have Juan and Angel been able to sustain such a lasting relationship in the face of HIV, illness, near death, infidelities, and new lovers? They say that what they're doing is "very un-American."

Angel explains, "My family takes it for granted I should take care of Juan, while my American friends bug me about it. Ecuadorian people say, 'Don't you dare leave Juan.' Americans say, 'Get rid of him. He costs you too much money.' "

"Juan has become my project. Ending the relationship has

crossed my mind. At times I get angry and frustrated. I have moments of rage, but then right away I have balancing emotions that
come and say, 'No, we'll be together forever until death.' "

"This has frustrated my boyfriend," Angel admits. "As long as
Juan is alive, my relationship with Kevin will never be normal. In
the beginning of our relationship, Kevin was expecting Juan to die.
Then it dawned on him that Juan would be around longer, and he
would have to adjust his way of thinking. I expected Juan to pass
within a year or two myself."

This is not unlike a phenomenon (described in Chapter 7) called
the "Lazarus syndrome," when people who expect to die don't.

"I made a commitment to be his caregiver forever, not his
lover," Angel continued. "I split out those roles. Until he can fly on
his own. He regressed during his illness, became like a child. He is
slowly coming back to being a man. He still doesn't have a job. I am
nurturing him. I'm not going to quit my project in the middle of it."

Can Men Nurture?:
Fighting Society's Values to Gain and Give Support

In selecting our partners and maintaining our relationships we have
to candidly look at the ability to receive as well as give support. By
its definition a relationship (as well as our health and that of our
partners) is something that needs ongoing care for it to succeed. As
gay men we are in the unique position to script our own rules when
it comes to the compassion and care we bring to one another and to
reject those that don't fit the parameters of how we see ourselves as
a couple.

NURTURANCE
VERSUS OVERDEPENDENCE

What is our ability to give and,
perhaps with more difficulty, receive nurturance? My work, especially with HIV-positive men, has
consistently shown that receiving
nurturance and care in their relationships is one of the greatest

> **As gay men we are in the unique position to script our own rules when it comes to the compassion and care we bring to one another and to reject those that don't fit the parameters of how we see ourselves as a couple.**

challenges for them. We are socialized to value independence and rugged individualism, and are educated as young children on the great statements about liberty and individuality in the Declaration of Independence and the Emancipation Proclamation. Nurturance—giving or receiving—may not come naturally to us. There is a conjecture that lesbian relationships tend to last in part because they are composed of two women, whom society has socialized to be nurturers. The implication is that men have not been so socialized.

Yet AIDS has brought gay men an opportunity to increase and centralize their role as nurturers within their relationships. AIDS has forced gay men to nurture themselves so as to remain HIV negative or stay healthy as people who are positive. It has required us also to care for our friends who become ill and die, and to comfort those left behind.

EQUALLY VALID AND EQUALLY NEGLECTED: BONDING AND SENSE OF COMMUNITY

It is not surprising in the context of this value system that the equally valid skills of bonding, understanding, and giving of self without losing the self are neglected and devalued. Affiliation and sense of community get lost when we are out of the neighborhoods and hometowns of an earlier age and as adults move into apartments where we don't know our neighbor's name but are fairly certain he has the same color of carpet in his living room and color of tile in his bathroom. Psychologist and author Jean Baker Miller, in her book *Toward a New Psychology of Women*, challenges the ideal of autonomy and recognizes that we perceive as feminine attributes and therefore devalue the skills of connection, attachment, and mutuality.[6]

However, AIDS has managed to create communities and the development of skills of affiliation for the gay/lesbian subculture, which then became a model for heterosexuals afflicted with HIV. Affiliation and our connection to others ensures the survival of self as well as peers. Alliances today can also be seen in the larger community, in the reported increase in volunteerism among younger generations of Americans, in the requirement that students perform community service to graduate from high school or the awarding of college credit for volunteer work done during a school semester.

The psychological model of healthy adulthood, for many, is one of growing as individuals and separating ourselves from our families. When and if we share our HIV status may be a contributing factor in moving away or growing closer to our families. Realizing that may not be an option for all of us or we may have to rely more on ourselves, our partners, and our own self-created families of choice and communities.

Striking a Balance: Helping versus Imposing

When I think about issues that come up as we progress through this disease and/or side effects of the treatments, I always recall a dear friend who eventually died of AIDS that I tried in vain to help. I offered and was willing to do some concrete and, for me, simple tasks that were difficult for him. Whether it was due to pride or politeness, however, he never accepted my assistance. His death left me feeling a little more empty, knowing I was not able to be there for him the way I had wanted to be. But I maintain respect for people's right not to have unsolicited assistance and protect their own privacy as they confront their illnesses.

The problem is that HIV as a disease almost always triggers fears in us about whether we will lose our autonomy and become dependent on others. The truth is that we probably will, in some way, become dependent. Circumstances may dictate that we will truly need the care and support of both professionals and friends at some point in the future. But will we become *overdependent*, which is what most of us mean when we use the word *dependent*? The American Psychiatric Association's *Diagnostic and Statistical Manual of Mental Disorders*, which is the bible for diagnosis, defines abormal dependence, such as that found in dependent personality disorder, as an "*excessive need* to be taken care of that leads to submissive and clinging behavior and fears of separation." Dependence that is pathological means "the difficulty in taking responsibility must go beyond what would normally be associated with [a serious general

> **HIV as a disease almost always triggers fears in us about whether we will lose our autonomy and become dependent on others.**

medical] condition or disability."[7] We need to find a way to recognize that relying on others for the things we can no longer do for ourselves, and that no one should be expected to be able to do, is not dependent in a disordered sense. It's just human.

THE CARE TEAM: A SMART ALTERNATIVE

One way to become more accepting if you are on the receiving end of help, or to offer it without imposing, is the care team. The premise of a care team is that often there are people in our lives who wish to be of assistance but do not know how to help and have their own fears of either being intrusive or overwhelmed. A care team is a group of people with differing skills, backgrounds, and time availabilities who are united in their desire to act as an extended family to someone who is seriously ill. When I proposed the concept, which is fully explained in the book *Share the Care*, by Cappy Capossella and Sheila Warnock,[8] to Jerry's friends, many of them expressed an interest and offered their skills:

"I'll be glad to walk your dogs for you."

"I'm always cooking too much food. I can bring over a pan of lasagna."

"I'm off every other Friday, and I'll be happy to spend it with Jerry."

I even received an offer for "help with the laundry."

All of these simple tasks can free up time for you to take care of other errands, sleep a little later, or know that you don't have to take the day off from work on a Friday. In the process, your partner may feel less guilty or fearful of overwhelming you, and meanwhile you can increase the level and quality of care for the person you love.

The process, described in the aforementioned book, is to call a meeting and explain that there may be some misgivings for a few members who lack a set of skills that maybe another team member has. Also for those positives who are single and ill, it provides a chance to have a different and unique intimacy that can occur within a caring context, to feel the closeness that takes place within the sphere of illness and active compassion.

Many AIDS organizations have recognized this concept in training people to be "buddies" for PWAs (people with AIDS) or to be other types of volunteer—good samaritanism which stems from people's desires to help. The trick for the HIV-positive person is to be open to this experience and realize it can be a blessing, which he can cherish and possibly enjoy. All the while those involved in your care grow in the process.

NURTURANCE FLUID AND RECIPROCAL

The care team contrasts with the traditional expectation—of the HIV-negative or healthier one giving to the HIV-positive individual—which does not recognize that nurturance can be mutual. From diagnosis/disclosure to later stages, caring still offers opportunities for an expression of nurturance that is fluid and reciprocal, versus a one-way and one-down model of compassion. "When Ben stopped working," said Andrew, age forty-four, "it was like having an old-fashioned relationship with a stay-at-home spouse. He cooked breakfast for me, took phone messages while I was at work, picked up the dry cleaning. He was still my equal, not devalued but revalued in different areas and different ways."

Often we, as positives, talk about our own spiritual and personal growth that occurs through this disease. If it can foster some of that in those around us, is there not a value and gift in that as well?

Autonomy or Sense of Connection?

Dr. Peter D. Kramer, psychiatrist and author of *Listening to Prozac*, a book on the effect of psychotherapeutic drugs on his patients' sense of self, questions in a later book, *Should You Leave?*, whether something is not lost in treating his patients' depression.

"Yes, the men and women attained relief, but perhaps something precious was lost in the process," Dr. Kramer wrote. "The issue was not only the means of transformation, but also the result. The very growth in autonomy that is such an overriding social good."

Moreover, Dr. Kramer notes, "Though not adept at tolerating isolation or demonstrating muscular self-esteem, some of the sensitive and generous men and women had their own genius. A genius for connection. Often they were romantic. They entertained impossible idealism. What medication offered them was autonomy, the ability to say no to others and attend to the self."[9]

Dr. Kramer, in this recent book, explores that question which is the most fundamental presented to therapists and the concurrent exploration of intimacy, autonomy, and advice.[10]

The Love Merry-Go-Round: Staying or Leaving

The definition of suffering according to Buddhist tradition is "clinging to that which changes." As we've described, for many couples HIV has acted as an emotional glue. But what happens when that is insufficient grounds for staying in a relationship? Making the decision to stay or leave when one or both partners has/have HIV can make it much more complex.

As we live longer with this virus, will we, as many couples do, outlive the value and purpose of our relationships?

Guilt and fear may cause tensions and the extension of an unsatisfactory relationship. As people live longer with this virus, will they, as many couples do, outlive the value and purpose of their relationship? The question of courage inevitably comes up here, as we consider whether we'll have the courage to work out some of the difficulties in a relationship or whether we'll believe we will survive the end of it.

A Lone Star: Alone In and Out of a Relationship

Deacon, as a survivor, has lived through hostility from the straight and the gay world: the tiny town in eastern Kansas where he was forced to remain closeted; homophobia from the military before he beat them at their own game; and his long stint as a gay bar owner where he experienced fraud and a forced buyout.

"I didn't know about gay people until I heard about them on the news. After that, I knew I was gay but didn't do anything about it until I resigned from the military. At that point I was about twenty-nine or thirty. During that time, I dated women, I even had a fiancée," he said. Being engaged to a woman is common among some closeted gay men. But Deacon took his hidden sexuality to an even deeper level. After he resigned from the U.S. Army, he served as a federal officer for the State Department, at which time he commanded a counterintelligence antigay squad during Desert Storm.

On the one hand, Deacon was in deep denial about his sexuality and was torturing himself by staying in that position. But, on the other, he knew these people were "family" he was being paid to witch-hunt and prosecute, and instead he acted to protect them.

Deacon always had business savvy, and he knew how to read the political climate in a professional situation so he could come out on top. How to beat the U.S. government at its own game? He actually used his position of power to protect gay people. "In two and a half years, not one homosexual was prosecuted. I protected them," he bragged.

He succeeded in rescuing these young soldiers, but will he be able to do the same for his own relationship? Deacon is at a loss and at a turning point regarding his relationship of nearly twenty years. Though his lover, Rod, has left him, Deacon is clinging to a relationship that is no longer there.

On a particularly frigid December night nearing Christmas, at a social in Washington, DC, I met Deacon in a group of HIV-positive men. I was drawn to this man who, with an appearance that spoke of another climate and culture, juxtaposed the weather and crowd 180 degrees.

He looked like a true transplant. Deacon is a cowboy. Tall, complete with Stetson hat, boots, and belt buckle, he stood as a loner in one corner of the hall and talked to me unabashedly about the loss of his true love. Deacon has HIV. His ex-lover has AIDS. Deacon is dealing with the emotions of loss before his friend is even dead.

Deacon met Rod in the late 1980s. Rod was a mere twenty-two years old, and Deacon was forty at the time. "I fell madly in love. He was intelligent, good looking. I thought all of this must come to him immediately, that he would know of his attributes," Deacon told me.

In and Out of Love

Deacon and Rod have traveled through every stage imaginable of a relationship. "We were in love, out of love, just roommates, friends, best buddies, family, brother, son and father, and then . . ." nothing? "Now it's hard again," Deacon says, not wanting to admit what might be the end.

But the commitment might have been over long before Rod officially ended it: "When we met, I was successful, he was jealous. He lived with me for four years and moved out when he wasn't getting everything he wanted. He was cheating on me, every other weekend he was gone. For the first two years I was totally faithful to him. We had major arguments, I threw him out five times, but he didn't have anyplace to go. Then I started sleeping with other people. For the last two years we lived together we were just roommates. When he finally moved out, I didn't want him to move out; he was like my son. I was dependent on him. There were no hard feelings, he just needed to go out and do his own thing."

"We maintained a close friendship. I would call him for advice; I trusted his opinion."

Through it all—from codependency to hot and steamy romance, which has now fizzled out to just being platonic friends—Rod has been Deacon's significant other.

Then a year ago, the bomb fell. At that time, Rod came to Deacon and said, "You have nothing I need." When asked why Rod would do such a thing, Deacon responded, "After all these years, he finally got a good job that paid him good money." But then the hidden, shameful truth surfaced. "At the same time, he told me he had tested positive."

Deacon continued, "I told him no big deal," for all this time Deacon had been dealing with his own HIV, and outside of getting extremely sick from experimental medication, he had never fallen ill directly from HIV. Deacon discovered in 1986 that he was positive, after the blood samples which were taken from him two years before were

TOO YOUNG TO TEST?

Even though the cases of AIDS in the United States have decreased since the early 1980s, it is reported that a lot of younger gay men who didn't live through many deaths of their friends from the disease currently are in denial—not getting tested, not using condoms, not getting treated.

Denial is an obvious reason. Many gay men feel that being positive is inevitable, so the longer they wait to be tested, the longer they can enjoy some level of comfort that denial and not knowing offers. While this reason for not testing might have been more valid before, with advances in current treatments, you pay a high price if you wait. Early detection can lead to highly improved conditions and longevity.

tested: "It showed I had the virus, but it was dormant. It stayed away for many years. Five to six years later, the symptoms came back."

Deacon continued, "I asked Rod for a T-cell count; he told me he didn't know it. A year before, he'd gotten real skinny but claimed he was negative. Then I discovered that for the past ten years he had lied. He never got tested" (see the box on the previous page).

"When I finally got him tested, his count was only 130. He had full-blown AIDS. I went into total shock. He apparently had been positive since the early eighties. He was positive before I met him," Deacon assumed. "But he would never accept the fact that he could have AIDS. We believe he knew he was exposed to AIDS in California, and had infected or reinfected dozens of people over the years."

The fact that Rod has left Deacon for good this time—not just physically, but emotionally—even as a friend, has Deacon stumped.

Was Rod really just using Deacon all these years and would have left Deacon once he got on his own two feet? Or is Rod now running due to his recent discovery of this potentially fatal disease?

Though Deacon is losing trust in any good they may have shared, deep down he suspects the most recent in a series of break-ups is due to HIV. "He used me to get what he wanted," he told me in one breath; but the very next breath brought "He can't accept help, he wouldn't accept it. I offered to pay his medical bills; he wouldn't accept that. He has awful insurance with his job. I tried to take care of him. He's still alive. He had pneumonia recently. But he's pushing me away, blaming me for all his failures."

One thing that kept them close before is the fact that Rod is estranged from his family. According to Deacon, Rod was raised by a neighbor. Deacon has been his family, and now Rod is rejecting him too (see the facing box).

Though Deacon says he's "not still in touch with him," he admitted that he had called Rod recently and asked how he was: "He was nice, then he got antagonistic. I think he has dementia. His personality has changed. He started getting weird two years ago—paranoid, argumentative—but his intellect wasn't affected. He now is like Jekyll and Hyde. Before he had a peaceful, loving, easygoing personality. I've had a hard time accepting he has dementia."

The More It Hurts, the Less It Works

Deacon has finally come to a point where he might consider the possibility that what he thought was a good relationship had

DEALING WITH ABANDONMENT FEARS

Here are some general guidelines for alleviating any fears of abandonment that are intruding on your relationships. You may find these measures more or less difficult to adopt. If you get stuck trying to implement any of the suggestions that you sense could help you, consult a therapist or counselor for assistance. For some of us, fears of abandonment are deep seated and will take some work to address:

1. Understand your childhood abandonment as well as past relationships where you blame someone for leaving you.
2. Monitor your feelings of abandonment. Identify your hypersensitivity to losing close people; your fears of being alone; your need to cling to people.
3. Be aware of uncommitted, unstable, or ambivalent partners even though they generate fireworks and excitement.
4. When you find a partner worthy of your devotion who is stable and committed to you, trust that he is there for you and will not leave.
5. Do not cling, become jealous, or overreact to the normal separations of a healthy relationship.

stopped working long ago, if it had ever worked. In her *Too Good to Leave, Too Bad to Stay*, Mira Kirshenbaum suggests looking at the best times of your relationship to see if they were really that good: "Some people, even in relationships that feel awful now, know that there was a time in the past when things were wonderful. They were in love, they were genuinely happy, they felt good about themselves when they were with the other—there was a kind of happy magic of warmth and connectedness. But other people realize that the 'best' was never very good. Something was wrong. They're usually referring to an empty, distant, tainted, painful quality at the core of their relationship, even back then."[11]

There were red flags at the beginning of Deacon and Rod's relationship. Rod was three hours late for their very first date and then moved to Boston, ostensibly because of a great job but actually, as Deacon later found out, to live with some other guy. It was only after Rod returned after a few months that he and Deacon ran into each other again and finally hooked up. And then there was the cheating and the presumed lying about HIV status.

When should someone pull the plug on a relationship?

Deacon and Rod had created a definition of their relationship that contrasts sharply with models based on consistency in monogamy, nurturance, or just overall availability. Still it persevered. Still it was permitted. And still Deacon wishes to be in it. Given their rocky history, I join Deacon in thinking this is not the end after all.

Rod, who may have not come to grips with his own illness, likewise has never been able to deal with Deacon's illness. "When I went to NIH [the National Institutes of Health] for experimental treatment of Interleukin 2 for the first time, Rod had moved out. The treatment caused me to be very sick for days—high fevers, nausea, dizziness, bloating, rashes. Rod was supposed to take care of me, but he showed up only one night even though at that time we were 'really close.' He was so screwed up, he wanted me to die. He told me that two and half years ago. At that time he didn't know he was positive also."

The icing on the cake is that Rod is currently dating someone Deacon was dating before he met Rod: "Over the years, this guy hated my guts because I dumped him. This guy hates me, Rod hates me. It is the essential 'fuck you' payback."

Deacon may attempt to blame all of Rod's nonnurturing behavior on dementia, but does Rod's past history bear this out?

After all is said and done, is the relationship over? It is unclear. "Rod is the only person I ever fell in love with," Deacon said. "I date now, I would love to have another relationship, but my love for Rod is so deep, I don't know if I can ever love someone again."

Till Death Do Us Part?

When do you have enough evidence that it is time to leave a relationship? Actually making a decision one way or the other is important to your mental, emotional, and physical health.

"If you've suspected that it's not good for you to stay up in the air, you're right. Staying ambivalent, in fact, can cause tremendous damage. Being stuck like this can end up killing you emotionally if you stay when you should be getting out. And it can end up killing your relationship if you keep thinking about leaving when it could be fixed if you only put energy into it. . . . And it's not as if waiting around is going to show you what's best for you. Ambivalence doesn't produce real answers. It's just a dangerous trap," wrote Kirshenbaum.[12]

So why didn't Deacon leave Rod long ago, and why is he still hanging on? Why do so many of us voluntarily experience this unnecessary pain?

Many of us were taught early in life that we will meet that one special someone who will take care of all our needs—spiritual, sexual, financial, and emotional—*till death do us part*. In reality, this can never happen; for our relationships to be healthy, we must take care of ourselves before we bring someone else into the love scenario. Believing the myth has prolonged many a relationship beyond its natural lifespan.

We also live in a culture that appears to value "relationships at all costs," a culture where people couple for status, one where being alone or single is looked down on.

Deacon may feel that leaving the relationship is admitting failure and that he has invested too much time and energy to give up. He is probably afraid of being alone.

As a social worker, I have worked with numerous couples over the years whose respect for each other has died, trusts were violated, or they had gone down such different paths that it was impossible for them still to have a "living, breathing relationship."

So ask yourself, what does "till death do us part" mean to you? If it means death of trust, death of caring and intimacy, then it is time to reevaluate your relationship.

By the same token, the physical death of a loved one can provoke similar types of clinging behaviors. In my work with clients who have a difficult reaction to loss, I introduce them to a different definition of suffering. Again, Buddhist philosophy defines suffering as

> **Ask yourself, what does "till death do us part" mean to you? If it means death of trust, death of caring and intimacy, then it is time to reevaluate your relationship.**

"clinging to that which changes." In other words, the longer you cling to something that is gone, the longer you will suffer. This grasping behavior lies at the root of much of the pain we experience during the ending of a relationship.

Hooked on Love

SIGNS OF RELATIONSHIP ADDICTION

1. Even though you know the relationship is bad for you (and perhaps others have told you this), you take no effective steps to end it.
2. You give yourself reasons for staying in the relationship that

are not really accurate or that are not strong enough to counteract the harmful aspects of the relationship.

3. When you think about ending the relationship, you feel terrible anxiety and fear, which makes you cling to it even more.
4. When you take steps to end the relationship, you suffer painful withdrawal symptoms, including physical discomfort, relieved only by reestablishing contact.

If most of these signs apply to you, you are probably in an addictive relationship. To move toward recovery, your first steps must be to recognize that you are "hooked" and then to try to understand the basis of your addiction. In this way, you can gain the perspective to determine whether, in reality, the relationship can be improved or whether you need to leave it.

WHEN TO SEEK PROFESSIONAL HELP

Some counseling may be called for when any of these four circumstances exist:

- When you are very unhappy in a relationship but are unsure of whether you should accept it as it is, make further efforts to improve it, or get out of it.
- When you have concluded that you should end a relationship, have tried to make yourself end it, but remain stuck.
- When you suspect that you are staying in a relationship for the wrong reasons, such as feelings of guilt or fear of being alone, and you have been unable to overcome the paralyzing effects of such feelings.
- When you recognize that you have a pattern of staying in bad relationships and that you have not been able to change that pattern by yourself.

Living and Loving Longer

As science progresses and lengthens our lives, so too will we experience the joy and challenges of being in longer-term relationships. Developing and strengthening the skills of caring and compassion will serve as a vital tool in preserving not only our physical health but the health of our relationships as well. The paradoxical benefit we also gain is the knowledge that the time we spend together comes from the conscious choice to stay in a committed relationship; it is that freedom of choice that binds us closer together than any other expectation or obligation can.

SEVEN

LAZARUS
AND SURVIVORS
Those Who Continue

For those of us who are survivors, whether unexpectedly living still with the virus or having outlived our partners, it is critical to our health to bring some sort of meaning to that role. Just as the discovery of your HIV-positive status can prompt change in your life, as discussed in Chapter 2, surviving your own near-death or your partner's death can bring adjustments.

Surviving bestows on us a new identity. Can you still be considered a person with AIDS (PWA) if you now have 400 T-cells and no apparent physical manifestation of illness? If you've lost your partner to AIDS, are you the same person you used to be now that you're not half of a couple? Survivors need to craft a new sense of self, and reestablishing a positive view of the world is integral to that process.

A 1998 study of forty HIV-positive men who experienced the loss of a partner showed that those men "who are prompted by the death of a loved one to make major shifts in their own values and priorities, emphasizing such things as close relationships, living each day to the fullest, and personal growth, may show physiological benefits, including a lower rate of mortality." The researchers found a difference of

---

Surviving bestows on us a new identity.

up to 155 T-cells between the men who made these shifts and integrated their grief and those who did not. This "discovery of meaning" and the deliberate contemplation of the loss increased the richness of the survivors' lives as well as the length of them.[1]

The survivors in this chapter have traveled to death's door. Some found the door shut; others watched as it closed on their partner and had to walk away alone.

Back from the Dead

His skin is smooth now with a healthy pink glow. His smile emanates from a clean-shaven, innocent baby face. His body frame is large, strong, and fit. Sitting in his kitchen, Gil told us the story of how just a few years ago a meeting with him would have taken place upstairs, where he had been bedridden. At that time his eyes were sunk into his head, his body was a skeleton, and he had grown a beard to cover the Kaposi's sarcoma (KS). "Every day I would prepare myself, thinking that it would be his last," Max, Gil's lover of fifteen years, told us. Considering Gil's current appearance, this was very hard for us to believe.

Gil exemplifies the *Lazarus syndrome*—a term coined to describe people with AIDS whose prognosis has been a sure and sudden death but who then metaphorically rise from the dead, recover, and find themselves among the living again. The syndrome is named for the brother of Mary and Martha of Bethany, whom Jesus raised from the dead (John 11:1–44; 12:1–11).

When Gil was sick, he had gone from 220 pounds down to 155. He's now at a healthy 186. He was bedridden for a year. At his worst— zero T-cells and a viral load of 1 million—he had more than eighty lesions covering his chest, legs, back, and face. His eyes were swollen shut most of the time. His body was wracked with undiagnosed rashes, the irritation from which could be relieved only by soaking in a tub full of scalding-hot water or burning them with a hair dryer.

Cursed and Blessed

Gil had the gamut of opportunistic and other diseases associated with "full-blown AIDS": *Mycobacterium avium* complex (MAC), internal and external KS, pituitary and thyroid disease, hypergonadism, neuropathy, and anemia. The worst was KS, he said: "I would wake up every morning with three new lesions."

Gil couldn't remember the exact year he tested positive. "It was 1990," Max reminded him. "Max is always correcting me," Gil said playfully. "I assumed I was positive for a long time since a guy I had been dating had died of AIDS. But I waited seven years before I got tested. I found out I was positive on my twenty-fifth birthday. I had a sore throat that wouldn't go away. When I went for a physical, my doctor suggested getting tested." That was seven years ago.

"After I was tested, there were two to three years of denial ," Gil continued. "Then, in September 1996, I got full-blown AIDS."

Max, now forty years old, has continuously tested negative. "I was more scared for Max than I was for myself," Gil said. "For the first three years of our relationship, we weren't having safe sex."

Throughout the worst period of his illness, Gil told us he was both cursed and blessed. Cursed because he belonged to what sounded like an atrocious HMO health insurance plan; blessed because he had the saintlike Max to take care of him.

"Gil was a very bad patient," Max finally admitted to us after skirting the issue for a while. We were interviewing the couple in the mocha-colored kitchen of their elegant Rockville house. Their house was spotless and formal. But in the kitchen there was a warm cozy feeling among us four as a cold winter rain poured down outside the window. Gil listened intently as Max, with a Tennessee accent, slowly re-created the story of how he was a "very bad patient," almost as if this were the first time Gil had heard himself described this way in such a forthright manner.

"He was angry with the entire medical profession," Max continued. "I had to make peace with his doctors every time Gil left an appointment, so he could go back to see them again." But then he retracted slightly: "Gil is a very sensitive person. He demanded that people do the best by him, and he didn't always get even 50 percent."

Gil did not disagree. "I had a very bad doctor. He was eventually fired for malpractice," Gil said. "His attitude was 'We'll keep you comfortable until you die.' He was a jerk and an asshole."

In support, Max added, "I would run him over with my car if I saw him."

"My doctor never even gave me a physical. He was a negligent person. There weren't a lot of doctors to choose from on my health plan," Gil explained. "On my HMO plan, the doctors were all in the same office, and they wouldn't allow a patient to go to another doctor in the same group. My advice to everyone is 'Pay more money than you think you should for good health insurance and do it while you're healthy.' "

In his hometown of New York, Gil eventually acquired another doctor whom his HMO did not cover. He also researched everything possible on HIV and entered medical studies to get the best possible medication.

"In the end, Gil got as good care as he would have gotten anywhere. He got himself out of bed. But the recovery he experienced, he did for himself. It was not what the doctors did for him," Max said.

For a long time, Max and Gil didn't think Gil would live from week to week, but they persevered with blind optimism. "We filled forms out ourselves, we entered the Crixivan lottery, and even passed up saquinavir, the first protease inhibitor on the market, because we were holding out for Crixivan, which is more powerful," Max said.[2]

Max quit his job as a software designer of five years to stay home and take care of Gil full-time for six months: "I wasn't considering myself or my future. I knew I would pick up my career at a later date. Gil needed a full-time nurse, and I wanted to stay near him. We cashed in on his life insurance policy, so we weren't worried about the money." Max has since switched careers.

"I never knew he was worried," Gil said of Max during that time period, even though Max admits now that he thought every day could be Gil's last. "All night long I would be incredibly thirsty, I didn't eat, I was in a semicomatose state, and I would ask him at 4 A.M. to get me something to drink, and he would get up, no complaints, and would just do it. I never saw him worry."

"I would give him little surprises, give him something to look forward to," Max said.

According to both Gil and Max, the illness has made their relationship stronger. Through the disease, they've learned how to get along much better. "Our relationship is so much more mature now," Max said. "Though we've only been together six years, it feels like a lifetime because of what we've gone through. We don't fight about stupid things anymore. I never once thought of leaving him, especially when he was sick. I made a commitment and plan to see it through."

Gil added, "I still can't wait to see him when he gets home from work. We're best friends. We eat dinner together every night like a family. We argue, but then we just kiss and make up."

This couple's strong commitment to each other could be one of the major factors that led to Gil's incredible recovery. After Gil was diagnosed as HIV positive, they went ahead and bought the house where they now live. "We were forging ahead anyway. We knew it [AIDS] would hit, but we didn't know it would be so soon," Max said. They bought the house eight months after diagnosis. Gil fell ill a year and a half later.

But Max was Gil's only constant emotional support throughout his illness. He was getting little help from the medical profession. Also, most of their closest friends deserted them, and they had to rely on people they knew a lot less intimately. Even Gil's family, while encouraging now, was of little emotional help (except for his twin) during the time Gil was most ill.

"His parents would come down occasionally, but it was sort of strange. His parents didn't even know Gil was gay until he first be-came sick," Max explained. "They had to accept his homosexuality and his disease at the same time. It took them a good year to accept it."

Ironically, Gil's father is a doctor, and his sister, Norma, is in medical research: "I had more expectations of my father. He was blindsided by this AIDS issue. All of a sudden, his son was dying of AIDS, and he couldn't help me, though he could have gotten me ac-cess to anyone, since his friends are the best scientists in the whole world. When I asked him for access, he would say he didn't know anything. That has changed since; now I get e-mails from him all the time with advice. I'm not angry at him anymore. I'm angry at my-self for not telling him sooner."

"I would have been in trouble if it had not been for Max," Gil concluded.

Of course Max is delighted that Gil has come back from the dead. But Max experienced an unexpected emotion, common among lovers of those who have come back to life. He felt angry when Gil recovered.

Max had been very stoic in his caregiving and had never even sought the comfort of a support group. "I don't believe in them. It wouldn't have changed what I had to come home to," he told us. Nor did he hold a grudge against the friends that had deserted them: "I just accepted it because I know that people are fickle." Yet Max was not quite as ready for Gil's recovery as he was for his death: "For years, I prepared myself to accept that he was going to die." The couple had a will made up and had been out searching for a cemetery plot. "I felt like the rug was pulled out from under me when Gil regained almost all of his strength," Max said. "I was angry for a couple of weeks. I felt like, 'Why was it necessary to put myself through this?' "

For individuals and couples who encounter what is now a more uncertain outlook as it pertains to health, the ability to plan, move forward, then back, and then forward again, requires the calling forth and expending of tremendous amounts of energy, which can manifest itself as anger when one becomes overwhelmed. In these cases, fear, exhaustion, and sadness can well up as anger.

But this may not be all bad. Anger, as a raw and now untargeted emotion, can be useful in mobilizing people into action. The positive use of well-delineated anger can be especially useful when we are dealing with hospital bureaucracies, insurance companies, and the occasional insensitive person we must encounter in the efforts of caretaking and survival. The flash of anger, especially in a protective manner toward an external threat, is an age-old way of expressing affection. Anger and affection are often paired in unlikely ways. We can experience a variety of forms of anger not only in our relationships but also in the situations that surround them, not all of which are negative.

In specific cases of the Lazarus syndrome, a caregiver who has spent much time and energy preparing for his partner to die, though relieved when he doesn't, may still feel like he wasted a lot of time preparing for the event. This might not make "logical" sense to the person experiencing the anger,

> **The positive use of well-delineated anger can be especially useful when we are dealing with hospital bureaucracies, insurance companies, and the occasional insensitive person one must encounter in the efforts of caretaking and survival.**

since much of this energy could very well have been critical in nursing his partner back to health.

A constructive method to deal with anger, one that has worked for my clients, is to talk about the feelings, no matter how horrible they seem or how guilty you may feel for having them. It is good to talk to a professional and/or peer counselor or support group, who can listen nonjudgmentally and not appear to be shocked or have a strong reaction to what you are saying. Talk to someone who listens and then repeats back your feelings and emotions, and who also probes, but with a few empathic questions. This interchange should allow you to vent and work through your feelings. You'd be surprised, but sometimes just hearing them out loud and confiding in someone you trust can bring a lot of relief.

Both Gil and Max have bounced back now and started new lives—better than the ones they had before Gil's near-death.

Gil never returned to his job in Maryland, where he ran a security firm. Instead, he has returned to school for his master's degree so he can teach—a dream he always had but never pursued—and produces a TV talk program on AIDS.

"When I was sick, I watched a lot of TV and only heard about AIDS through negative sound bites. I thought to myself then that if I ever got better, I would learn how to do television and would put something out there that people can check into. So I now host a weekly talk show."

Max emotionally supports Gil during times of self-doubt, when Gil is tempted to go back to his old job. "Max encouraged me to do it [go back to school]. More than once I wanted to go back to work, and he said 'No. Take a second chance from life. I would.' "

Max has returned to the working world full time but has chosen another career path, which he likes better than software development.

Even though Gil is feeling much better now, he still has a lot of maintenance problems that aren't presently repairable. He still has KS and MAC infection that will require treatment for the rest of his life. This is a reminder that he is still vulnerable to the constant threat of illness, though Max is more optimistic. "We've already lived the worst. We don't have to relive that again," Max said. "I don't think this disease will kill Gil; he's too determined to beat it."

But Gil doesn't necessarily believe that: "HIV is too sneaky a disease. I don't trust it."

Headlines and Hope

This was supposed to be the last time the AIDS Memorial Quilt would be seen in its entirety. With the Quilt rolled out on the Mall in Washington, DC, and the Washington Monument in the background, the fall of 1996 seemed like an optimistic time for this final viewing.

Three months earlier, in July, the Eleventh International Conference on AIDS in Vancouver, Canada (the same summer as the Olympics in Atlanta), brought with it the excitement, the hype and hope for a cure. It was an opportunity to rebuild, to brush aside with pills and potions this illness that had sent us to the dry cleaner to press suits and formal attire worn more often to funerals than to weddings.

My partner and I were featured in three front-page stories of major newspapers. One headline read, "I Never Thought I'd Live to Forty." The story goes on to describe how Jerry had spent two weeks in the hospital and I was told to start preparing for the end.[3]

But surprisingly, that October Jerry returned to his job as an attorney for the U.S. Department of Justice, and the newspaper story went on to describe how he had "unretired" off "permanent disability."

The return to work was a scary process for both of us. Having done some of the emotional preparation for death, either individually or as a couple, the prospect of resuming a new and unplanned-for life could have been either a wonderful experience or one filled with trepidation. We were sprinters training for the hundred-yard dash now switched to competing in a marathon—eager to take up the baton, believing still we would see the finish line.

AIDS, up until that point, had been a logical and predictable disease. Get tested, get sick, go on disability, and die. Of course, there were exceptions: those who were called "long-term survivors" (later the term was changed to "nonprogressors") and those who were diagnosed on their deathbeds.

In the aftermath of the Vancouver conference there was an attempt by the medical profession to rewrite the script, making the ending—of the virus or our lives as we knew them—less certain.

With newly monogrammed shirts his mother had bought for him, Jerry went back to work. The first Christmas after his return, CNN did an interview with us. Meanwhile, *Time* magazine named David Ho their 1996 Man of the Year for his research involving the new "miracle" drugs, protease inhibitors. CNN filmed a special on the drugs, which featured a success story: my partner, Jerry. A year later CNN did a follow-up: this time they filmed a memorial service and images of me, alone, decorating the Christmas tree that Jerry had ordered four months before.

Jerry became the poster boy for the Lazarus phenomenon by returning to work and allowing the media to follow his progress. With this, came a new anxious hope from all of us—a hope that was to be strong enough to keep Jerry alive and be a new type of hero in this epidemic—one who survived. I was assigned a visible role as the supportive spouse. An effort that I had heretofore conducted in private was now making national news. The experience of losing a loved one (after the drugs failed Jerry) ended as a *Washington Post* front-page story that we shared with the headline announcing the death of Princess Diana.

Little did we know then that soon we would be confirming an old science writer's axiom that any new medical treatment can be guaranteed to generate two headlines. The first is "Treatment X is a Miracle Cure"; the second, a year or so later, is "Dangers of X Revealed"—or (in the case of AIDS) "Many Still Lose the Battle."

During our media coverage, Jerry's story of taking the "miracle" drugs soon took on the last headline.[4]

The same weekend the Quilt was in town in its entirety, memorializing those who had fallen, Jerry was receiving the Whitman–Walker Clinic's Courage Award because he had risen and was returning to work and to the promise and responsibilities of life. In receiving that award he symbolized a hope that the end of the disease was near. In the sunlight that badge of courage did look gold. Now I am careful not to polish it too thoroughly lest I find bronze.

Will It Last?

But courage cannot exist without fear.

As a child, I enjoyed the Saturday afternoon horror movies filled with those who had come back from the dead—Dracula, Frankenstein's monster, armies of zombies. So not surprisingly, I began to see in my therapy practice and in my relationship those expressions of fear and uncertainty in response to this eradicated foe. They were played out in questions like: How long will this new life last? What about side effects? Will I be forced to go back to work? Will my insurance cover the treatment—and, if not, can I afford it?

These and other questions and concerns surfaced as a counter-weight to the declining number of obituaries we saw in our local papers. For many of my clients and peers, preparing for death meant running up credit cards, partying a little harder, living *for* the moment versus living *in* it. With a new lease on life the credit card bills came due and the occasional cocktail or snort of cocaine turned into suggestions from friends that you think about getting help. The privileges and rights that the seriously ill may claim or that are allotted to them began to diminish as these new drugs started to work. Contributions and attendance at AIDS organizations' fund raisers were down. People were tired of AIDS. It was now passé (see the box).

As CNN followed Jerry back to work, I could still hear beneath his monogrammed shirts the whirring of the small engine that pumped the medicine to keep in check his cytomegalovirus (CMV) so he wouldn't lose his eyesight. It also pumped a drug we jokingly called amphoterrible (amphotericin B) to keep his thrush in check and which often caused him to shake uncontrollably with chills. These and other fluids were sent to the port in his chest to keep him sufficiently hydrated and to fight off infection.

> Andrew Sullivan, former senior editor of *The New Republic* and the author of *Love Undetectable,* wrote a piece for the *New York Times Magazine* titled "When Plagues End." He stated, "A difference between the end of AIDS and the end of many other plagues: For the first time in history, a large proportion of the survivors will not simply be those who escaped infection, or were immune to the virus, but those who contracted the illness, contemplated their own deaths and still survived."[5]

I also remembered how the children in the book *Little House on the Prairie* had kept baked potatoes in their pockets to keep their hands warm and from this got the idea to microwave whole potatoes and apply them to the parts of Jerry's body that I couldn't cover with mine when his chills were the worst. I remember him still weakly smiling with temporary relief.

Hope Unfulfilled: Grief Returns

Jerry's doctor's visits continued after he went back to work. The optimism carried us through. Then a return to the hospital. The monogrammed shirts hang limply in the closet now.

ANTICIPATORY GRIEF

"Grief is the phenomenon encompassing the mourning, coping, interaction, planning, and reorganization that are stimulated and begun in part in response to the awareness of the impending death of a loved one and the recognition of anticipated losses in the past, present, and future. It mandates a delicate balance among the mutually conflicting demands of simultaneously holding on to, letting go of, and drawing closer to the dying loved one."

—Theresa A. Rando, *Loss and Anticipatory Grief*[6]

I hesitate and question the tone of my own voice in speaking about his and my own struggle with the illness (see the box on anticipating grief). Having tasted the sweetened promise of a return to life only to have my own grief process reactivated, I don't want to sound bitter while looking at pharmaceutical ads for protease inhibitors that show men climbing mountains or throwing javelins. I remember the health warnings on another chemical wonder, which was first advertised as a healthier substitute for sugar. Is hope now being repackaged as was saccharine, which was later linked with cancer in laboratory rats?

The Questions of Survival: What Now and How Long Will It Last?

For the biblical Lazarus as well as the modern ones, coming back can cause unexpected complications. What does coming back mean? How will roles change now that the couple's vision for the future has altered dramatically? Did Lazarus come back an old Jewish man? Did his wife have her eye on some nice young Jewish man while he was sick? And what are the limits of new drug treatments? To what extent can they restore health?

The "Protease Moment": Believing and Beginning

What Eric Rofes (author of *Dry Bones Breathe: Gay Men Creating Post-AIDS Identities and Cultures*) called the "protease moment" has reset many biological clocks.[7] As we live longer, we will take the risks the living take, versus the risks taken by those who believe they may die.

Couples living in the protease moment may reexamine their relationships and either develop the tools for a longer haul or contemplate leaving their relationship. Believing in their new lease on life, they may feel they have the strength to exit a relationship, bring new meaning to it, or even begin a new one.

Many men, as they attempt to reengage their lives, realize that these protease inhibitors have given them the freedom to pursue new jobs—and perhaps new boyfriends as well. Jason, a friend of mine, described the midlife crisis he never expected to face: and the need to be found sexually attractive despite growing older: "I feel like he just saps my energy—when I was ill he was there for me, but now that I feel better that stability I craved and needed then makes him appear more blah, less exciting."

This creation of a new and improved identity is reminiscent of the behaviors I had seen in those recently diagnosed HIV positive. Realizing that time was short, these men felt they should straighten their lives out. Jason and others were having a similar response to having their lives extended rather than cut short: reexamining their lives and how they intended to live them.

In some ways—dare I say it?—I am secretly excited that someone with HIV can now contemplate leaving a safe but emotionally and sexually unfulfilling relationship. When you perceive yourself as dying, your heart calendar and stopwatch may not allow time to contemplate a breakup, closure, dating, and possibly falling in love again. Those are the homework assignments of the living. Jason must now answer the question that all Lazaruses ask: "What do I do now?"

It's natural to take advantage of a new lease on life. But what about these men's partners? Committed to them, they have held on to the belief that the only way their relationship would end would be when their lovers died in their arms. Now the specter of a different kind of ending has been raised, and of course many of these men feel betrayed.

As we noted at the end of Chapter 6, living longer also presents opportunities to love longer, which creates new challenges. Jason knows he will be around longer, which brings the unanticipated dilemma of starting and adjusting to a new job,

> **When you perceive yourself as dying, your heart calendar and stopwatch may not allow time to contemplate a breakup, closure, dating, and possibly falling in love again.**

and he is contemplating being single again. Just as many of us may have rushed to the belief, immediately after our HIV test results came back positive, that imminent death, doom, and destruction loomed on the immediate horizon, we must be cautious of making drastic changes now that current treatments offer a new optimism.

In my role as social worker, I focus with these men on their transition of returning to work and stress the advantage of having a somewhat predictable and reliable partner during a major life change. We take the energy generated by their enthusiasm and hope and increased physical health and well-being and focus it on one major life task at a time—in this case a new job. Building on the confidence they might gain in this achievement, they can then decide if they are ready to end their current relationships. Then we contemplate the risks and rewards of being single again and the impact that would have on their current partners, whom I encourage to join us in the event they want to move forward with a breakup. For many men, starting a new job may require that we meet a few more times to discuss this transition, and some then decide that for now they want to maintain their relationships.

While some men never return to my office, what I see now, as a therapist working with gay men, is that I rely more on the skills of a couple therapist, as a mediator and negotiator, and less on those of a grief counselor, when it comes to the question of how and if their relationship will end. In this way, I am finding relief and satisfaction in how my work is evolving and changing just as my patients' lives are.

The Practical Challenges of Staying Well

Deciding how to take advantage of the gift of survival is a momentous task, to be certain, and can involve many emotional choices. But those who are experiencing the Lazarus syndrome have to face certain practical challenges as well. Staying well isn't easy and sometimes brings unexpected problems.

The protease inhibitors have given us increased hope and vitality, but there is a downside that may be difficult to detect through the rose-colored glasses that often come with the Lazarus syndrome.

As I acted on my decision to add a protease inhibitor to my regimen, for the first time since being diagnosed I felt physically unwell. The side effects—most notably gastrointestinal—made me realize that there was a price to be paid for a possible extension on life.

More broadly, I realize that I have not been cured and can still transmit the virus. What too often has been called the "War on AIDS" now feels to many of us like an uneasy truce. Yes, many of us have beaten death, at least for the time being. But returning to work and trying to resume a more routine life bring their own problems, because we remain ill—we just aren't progressing as quickly.

New services are appearing to respond to the unique needs of this now healthier population of HIV-positive individuals. AIDS service organizations are going into new areas of treatment: vocational rehabilitation, job placement assistance,

What too often has been called the "War on AIDS" now feels to many of us like an uneasy truce.

and increased funding for these costly drugs. AID Atlanta, for example, that city's oldest AIDS service agency, has designed a program to help clients cope with their emotions. The counseling program, called Reconstruction, leads patients through topics like "Hype versus Hope" and "Wake Up and Smell the T-Cells" in an effort to ease what Mark King, the program coordinator, called "a return to the rat race."

If AIDS once seemed like a relentless descent downhill, it's now a roller coaster—of health, illness, then maybe health and illness again, and (we hope) one day recovery. We spend increased and unexpected time in health and recovery when the drugs work, and we spiral downward into anger and resentment when they don't. Those who are partnered with us and are acting as caretakers have to ride the roller coaster too, from hope to dread and back again.

The uncertainty of the "new" AIDS has had obvious benefits: a decline (at least currently) in AIDS deaths and in the number of patients seen for treatment of opportunistic infections. But it has had unexpected negative consequences: an increase in the number of the HIV-positive who experience anxiety, depression, and—surprisingly—suicidal thoughts.

Do the Lazaruses of the world feel some urge to reset their own biological clocks to fulfill a destiny they once thought was immutable? Maybe so. A 1998 *New York Times* article reported: "The Lazarus syndrome is unique to HIV and AIDS, with no easy parallel to other illnesses. 'Perhaps the closest comparison is to the trauma suffered by people from German concentration camps,' said Dr. Linda Moneyham, a researcher at the University of South Carolina, who is studying the phenomena. 'Like many people with AIDS who got very sick, Holocaust survivors watched their families and friends die, and fully expected to follow, but instead were suddenly freed to a precarious and lonely world.' "

" 'It all boils down to uncertainty,' Dr. Moneyham said. 'Sometimes even though the known is bad, at least you know what it is and you know what to do about it.' "[8]

Perhaps this explains why some people have been seen to attempt a sort of passive suicide, where they underdose themselves or stop taking their medication altogether. This form of self-destructive behavior has a different quality from more aggressive approaches like taking an overdose of pills. But it's the latter that we clinicians are trained to expect. So at the hospital where I worked, we began to ask patients about their medication compliance to identify those who were experiencing some sort of suicidal thoughts.

Even as Jerry was returning to work and Bret was considering leaving his partner, I was also making major life decisions within the context of the promise of these new drugs for Jerry. Feeling confident about Jerry's health, I decided to leave the safety of a government job doing HIV prevention work and return to full-time clinical work.

Beginning this new job meant I would not immediately have access to the vacation and sick leave time that I had used frequently to take Jerry to the hospital or accompany him to his varied outpatient appointments and procedures. To be sure, many appointments were more or less routine; however, the first time he received an injection in his eye, placement of a new catheter, or a drilling in his back hip bone for a marrow sample I made it a point to be there and luckily had a supportive workplace that allowed me to leave early some days or take longer lunch breaks.

Within a year of Jerry's return home and seeming remission, I was touring a hospice with his mother, preparing for his death. Then, two days before he died, Jerry perked up and seemed to improve in energy, appetite, and outlook. I was briefly concerned that perhaps I had been premature in calling his family to fly out to Washington, DC, from Nebraska. He soon relapsed, however.

Holding his hand, surrounded by his parents and brother, before he quietly exhaled his last breath, I told him how beautiful he looked (though he had had a seizure shortly beforehand and had tubes in his arm and chest). That was the way he appeared to me. Afterward, I took the flowers we had brought him, crumpled them in a basin of warm water, and bathed his now lifeless body. One last intimacy I would have with his body but not with his spirit (see the box).

Jerry Roemer was supposed to be the new face of AIDS.

For a few fleeting, joyful months last winter, Mr. Roemer was strong and vital. Though he had been infected with HIV for years, the amount of deadly virus in his blood had plunged by 98 percent, the result of a powerful cocktail of new drugs called protease inhibitors that brought him back from the brink of death.

After two years on disability, he returned to his job as a lawyer for the Department of Justice, happily informing colleagues that he had "unretired." Attorney General Janet Reno called him an inspiration. His parents kept their fingers crossed; for Christmas, they bought him monogrammed shirts for work.

On Wednesday, Jerry Roemer was buried in a graveyard surrounded by cornfields near his family's Nebraska farm. He spent his final days in a seventh-floor room at Georgetown University Medical Center, a skeleton of the handsome man he once was. . . .

"It wasn't supposed to happen this way," Mr. Roemer said one afternoon when he felt well enough to speak. The next evening, encircled by his parents and brother, his partner and his doctor, he died. He was 32.[9]

Copyright New York Times, August 22, 1997

Optimism Kept Him Alive: The Story of Burt

His eyes and cheeks are partly sunken, a baseball cap is on his head to hide hair loss from chemotherapy, KS scars are on his arms under his sweatshirt, and he dons large baggy sweatpants to hide excessive swelling. But when I met him Burt was still the picture of health, at least emotional health. And his eyes were twinkling and flirtatious.

"I'm in the ugly ducking stage and waiting for the swan act," he tells me with humor, but he is serious. Only one week out of the hospital and he is lining up dates—tomorrow is dinner with a friend. "I've been craving lobster, and I think I should have it," he tells me.

He reclined on his couch in his modest one-bedroom apartment in northwestern DC as his mother, who flew up from Texas and has been tending him since he became deathly ill this last time, rests in the next room.

His mother, a small Mexican woman, met me at the door and served me homemade Christmas cookies and brewed a strong pot of coffee before she retired to the bedroom at 9:00 P.M. A small decorated Christmas tree adorned one corner of the living room, a tree that his mother and sister had decorated for Burt while he was in the hospital. Even his family was hopeful of his return. It was only a week and a half until Christmas and one of the colder nights we'd had in DC that winter.

Burt almost died twice. Once in 1995 in a Boston hospital, from PCP (*Pneumosystis carinii* pneumonia), and the last time in a DC hospital only a week before I interviewed him.

"I should be dead. But I'm still here! Isn't that shocking?" he asked me with genuine enthusiasm and disbelief.

"This last time I thought I was going to die. I didn't think I could pull it off. I even thought about calling a priest to read me my last rites.

"But now I think I'll last forever. Either die of old age or get hit by a bus. But I could go at any time. I got sick so fast over Thanksgiving."

Reinventing Himself

Burt says the way he's staying alive is by reinventing himself over and over. He started this process way before he was diagnosed. He traced it back to age 18, in Corpus Christi, Texas, when he changed his last name, which was Spanish, to a typically Anglo name, trying to survive and separate himself from his lower-socioeconomic Mexican upbringing. His family was large with little education. Both his parents and some siblings are alcoholics, but there is a lot of love and closeness all the same. His mother has traveled to stay with him both times he nearly died.

As an HIV-positive adult and now forty years old, he has reinvented himself the same way to avoid a death sentence of AIDS.

Storing away the once inevitable diagnosis of death in another part of his mind, he has stayed busy, volunteering at his job, dressing well, investing his life insurance money in the stock market, and collecting pop art.

The oldest of nine children, and considered the independent, strong "hero" in the family, since 1993 Burt has been fighting a progressive case of KS that swells his legs and groin up to incredible sizes. "I'm the overachiever, the golden fleece of the family, a Scorpio," he says. At one point he could hardly walk, couldn't fit into any of his clothing, weighed 240 pounds; his scrotum was as big as a grapefruit, and he couldn't lace up his shoes. And during all of this, he kept pushing. In the dead of winter in Boston, he would find a way to dress himself, get on a bus, and go volunteer at Rep. Joe Kennedy's office, the job from which he had to retire. Or he would bundle up and walk down the street to a coffee house, to distract himself from his disease, while his mother became hysterical and worried about his health.

Burt believes he is still alive from sheer will. He has watched the other seven people who were in his Taxol experimental drug study for KS die. He is the only survivor. And after his first bout with pneumonia in 1995, the doctors gave him only a few weeks to live, a few months at best:

"My doctors said they didn't expect me to survive. My mind never gave in to that thought. I never gave up. I kept very busy. The physicians said mine was a terminal condition. I separated that into one part of my brain and kept going.

"At one point I thanked my doctor for keeping me alive, and he told me, 'Burt, you're doing so well because of the way you live your life, your attitude. It's not me.' It's true, because I knew I was a goner, but I never allowed it to sink in."

Burt had a long haul to get to this level of perseverance. After he was first diagnosed in 1993, by what he described as an insensitive doctor, he went into denial for a few months, didn't tell anyone, and didn't seek out health care.

After discovering a spot on his arm, his HMO doctor, who didn't think it was HIV, sent him to a dermatologist, who after seeing the spot, shrieked, "Oh, my God!! When is this going to stop??? How do you feel?? You have Kaposi's sarcoma!!" She then insisted on informing the surgeon who was going to remove the cyst on his back that it was now KS and that he had HIV.

His original HMO primary care doctor exclaimed after he

found it was indeed KS, "I'd have to go through a bunch of loops to get you on chemotherapy," which he never did. He only gave him a prescription for AZT and dismissed him. Burt believed the AZT made him ill, and he never took it again.

Meanwhile, Burt had been working for Rep. Joe Kennedy in his Capitol Hill office for three years, after he had worked in Kennedy's home office in Massachusetts for four years. His career was going well as special assistant to Kennedy, but his body was ballooning up due to the edema and he was trying to ignore it.

"Everyone in the office was talking about me behind my back, and I wanted out of the office." Burt applied to the U.S. Department of Labor for a position, got hired on the spot, and saw this as his great escape from "his friends in the office." But when it was time to resign, Joe Kennedy took him aside, told him he wished he wasn't quitting, and asked, "By the way, how's your health?"

At that point, Burt broke down, told Kennedy he was HIV positive, and sobbed. Kennedy held him in his arms and convinced him to move back to Boston, where he could work in the home office with less pressure, and he would set him up with some of the finest AIDS specialists in the country.

Fighting to Live

This was the beginning of Burt's fight to live. He did move to Boston, hooked up with one of the AIDS research pioneers and a KS guru, was one of the first to take the cocktail Crixivan, and one of the first to take Taxol for KS. He also decided to go on Social Security disability, collected $300,000 from his life insurance, took a wellness course, joined support groups, and took up scuba diving when his health returned.

Burt has always considered himself a fighter. "I didn't have money when I was growing up or in my early adulthood, but I was very bright and used my beauty as an asset," he told me. "It opened up a lot of doors for me. I survived death by constantly reinventing myself. I grew a goatee, collected art. I learned how to dress, became a master illusionist. I learned that if I wore dark pants I could hide the swelling."

One of Burt's art pieces in his growing collection loomed behind him on the living room wall. The piece is by Paul Richard and is a photo of Burt and his sister in South Boston, taken on some railroad tracks in the wind. The work symbolizes parts of Burt's life. "It's a family portrait," he explained. Many books are scattered on the tracks, to represent Burt's extensive library; he is holding the *New York Times*, which he religiously reads every day; and his sister, a major support system for Burt, sits on a rickety chair in the background. "The photo is taken on an angle so you can't see my swelling that much," he explained.

He now considers himself part of the Lazarus phenomenon, especially after this last time in the hospital, where he had a series of dreams, all having to do with experiencing death and returning from it:

"I had dreams of going into pools of water, feeling the smoothness of it, and going deeper, deeper, deeper. It felt good to be in the water. But then I resisted and came back out of the water. Another dream I was fighting flash floods and trying to protect myself from the water while I was barely clothed."

Though he wards off death with a strong resolve, he has prepared for death in many ways: he has a living will; he has readied a burial plot and arranged for a coffin in his home town of Corpus Christi; he has bequeathed his art collection to a museum in his home town, to be later turned over to his family; he has decided who is to receive 180 autographed collectible books; and he has written friends to tell them how much they have meant to him, in the event that he passes. His head is not completely in the sand when it comes to his longevity. While he does plan for that possible unfortunate end, he spends the rest of his time planning for the future.

Yet, he didn't always have an easy time being mentally positive. He described himself as being on a "death wish" while living in Boston: "My friends were dying. My world was getting smaller. I came out to friends as having AIDS and lost many friends, gay and straight. I became more promiscuous and starting drinking more, doing more drugs. I was too ashamed to take off my clothes with any dates because of the KS, so I started using an escort service. I hated it. I moved back here a year ago to try to get away from all that."

Since he's been back, except for this last bout with pneumonia (PCP), Burt feels that things are looking up for him.

Now, "the initial trauma has become just a way of life—dealing with AIDS."

Dealing with the Guilt

*You never know what is enough until you know what is
more than enough*

—William Blake

Surviving your partner often brings guilt. People left behind may
ask themselves, "Did I do enough to keep him alive as long as possible? Did I let my own burden and needs get in the way of taking
care of my spouse? Why did he die instead of me? Or instead of a
hundred and one other people who do not have as much warmth
and compassion as my lover had? Surely those people are more worthy of death and pain than my partner was."

These questions, which are impossible to answer, can delay us
from moving on with our lives and eventually getting over the loss.

People deal with grief in many different ways: some deny it;
some drown it out in destructive or obsessive behaviors; some
throw themselves into another relationship right away, postponing
inevitable pain; others move through it healthily.

Consider the following story of how someone moved past regret and sorrow.

Crystal Balls and Computer Screens: Contacting the Dead

Milo is a fifty-year-old insurance actuary, HIV negative, and someone whom I have known for years through a mutual hobby. He got
past the pain and guilt of surviving his lover, Vince, by accessing an
unconventional source.

Vince's death was a difficult one—for both Vince and Milo. Before Vince died, he had an advanced case of dementia caused by
CMV spreading to his brain, which led him to lash out in violent episodes, and he suffered from wasting syndrome. He was also refus-
ing help from Milo.

"It wasn't him," Milo explained.

On top of that, Vince lived in a basement apartment in an im-
poverished neighborhood and at the time of his illness was living
off a poor man's pension he was receiving from a supermarket
chain for which he had operated a fork-lift for a decade.

Milo lived in a classy loft apartment in a better part of town,
where Vince refused to visit, for fear of "messing it up," since he

had become incontinent. Staying over at Vince's wasn't an enticing idea for Milo, since the heat had been turned off in Vince's apartment and he was living in the bedroom with a kerosene lamp. Vince needed to be hospitalized, but Milo didn't have medical power of attorney. He was waiting for Vince's nephew, a lawyer, to finagle the papers so that Vince could receive unsolicited help. Milo said, "He was like a homeless man in his apartment. I stopped going there. I wanted to get Whitman–Walker Clinic and Food and Friends in there to help, but he wouldn't let me. He wouldn't even let me pay the gas bill."

All this was too much for Milo. Milo also felt strongly that Vince really wanted to die and that Milo's presence was preventing him from doing so. So he left for two weeks—went to Manhattan and milled around in a daze, and then went to visit his mother in Florida. While he was in Florida, Vince passed. Milo found out through a phone call. Vince was found by a good friend, a neighbor, lifeless, sitting on top of his bureau. Even though Milo knew Vince was near the end, maybe even wanted him to pass at this point, he had regrets:

"Vince was a poor man, but I loved him with all my heart. We were together five years, and we didn't live together. I've been thinking about it, and I've been having regrets about letting old relationship fears not let me go to another level. He would have lived with me. By the time I started thinking I would want to, it was too late. He was real sick by then."

Milo also felt bad about not taking care of Vince full time: "I couldn't be there all the time. Sometimes I felt uncomfortable being there. I wanted him to come here. The guilt started to get to me. Benny, his nephew, lived upstairs, and he had a friend across the street look after him. It was a three-pointed caregiver team.

"The last two weeks of his life, I knew he was coming to the end. Patty, his nurse, confirmed for me it was the end. She said he had only three weeks, a month left. I knew that Vince was anxious to leave, and he needed me to be away because I wasn't letting him go. I wouldn't let him die. I would say, 'I don't want you to die.' He would say, 'We don't have much choice.' I knew if I stayed on the scene, he wouldn't be able to leave.

"For the first few months, I dealt with a lot of guilt for going away and knowing full well that it was the thing that got him to Glory."

Milo spent the year after Vince's death in heavy grieving. Burying his head in Vince's clothes he had held on to, weeping for hours. Blaming himself for not being there when Vince actually died. Keeping a "shrine" for Vince throughout the apartment of pictures and assorted bric-a-brac.

Then something happened that dissolved Milo's guilt.

About a year after Vince died, Milo contacted a woman over the Internet who helped him get over Vince by "contacting the dead." Milo just happened along a now defunct site on the Internet called *afterdeath.com* where people shared their grief over losing loved ones. He posted a message, exchanged e-mails with others in grief, one of whom referred him to a woman in California who offered three-way "conference calls" with the person who is grieving, the dead person, and herself, for a fee.

Milo decided to do it.

"This twist of events resolved the guilt," Milo told me. "This lady could transcend to another realm of existence: talk to dead people. A friend of mine had gotten together with her dead brother, and the experience had lifted her into another state of consciousness when she found out he was in a place where he was well and thriving."

"We decided that the night of December 15 would be my 'discernment' night—to have a reading. We did it over the phone. For about four to five days in advance I was told to talk to Vince to alert him of this meeting. During the phone call I had his picture next to me, with his favorite music—Motown oldies—playing in the background. While we talked, the revelation started coming to me. While she was describing what she was experiencing, I knew Vince was who she was with. I started weeping right there. I knew it was him. She said his death was peaceful, he just slipped away. Exited stage left. She said I was being too hard on myself. That Vince said I did a good job taking care of him, that he didn't know if he'd do such a good job if the tables had been turned. I got a lot of reassurance that he was well and happy.

"The discernment provided the closure I needed, helped me move on. I met Jesse, my new lover of one year, five days after my discernment."

Jesse is HIV negative, and they are "moving slowly, but in a direction that will take us to another level—living together," Milo said.

"That's what I really want. Vince would tell me he wanted me to meet somebody and move on with my life."

One picture of Vince remains on Milo's "family photo" wall. Vince, an older man, graying hair, peeks out with a bashful smile, while dressed in soft-looking overalls and posed in front of a wall of cartons next to his fork-lift.

From Stripper to Activist: Grief and Transformation

Michael's guilt acted itself out in two chapters. Immediately after his lover, Steven, died, he dove into a relationship that he describes as "not being very constructive. It was only later when I ditched that relationship that I started dealing with these unpleasant feelings in a healthy way," he said.

Eleven years ago, when Steven died, Michael buried the guilt and pain in a relationship with a married man, only five months after Steven's death:

"I felt guilty that he was sick and I wasn't. He had a career, I didn't. He was an engineer, the 'golden boy,' the only boy in his family. His father had died. His mother hoped he would carry on the family name. If he hadn't met me, he would have found a nice Jewish woman to be with, his mother used to say. He had more to live for than I did. Why did he get sick and I didn't? I was just as trashy [Michael, who is HIV negative, had shared needles with Steven]. I was angry at myself. We weren't monogamous. I was having [safe] sex outside the relationship."

"I haven't been in a normal relationship since then," Michael continued. "It scares me. I don't want to end up being the bachelor uncle like a lot of gay men in their forties and fifties. Sex is easy to get, but there is no romance. I believe in romance. Maybe I'm not allowed to have anyone else [besides Steven]."

Getting involved with a married man meant that Michael didn't have to be so committed, that he didn't completely do a disservice to his lover's memory. It also meant, however, that he didn't have to deal with being alone.

"Steven died in February 1987. I was dancing in a bar for a living, and I met someone at the club that summer. He was married. I stayed in the relationship; I was with him for seven years. The sex was good. He was ten years older than me. He would come here once a week. I wanted someone to latch on to. I wasn't ready for anything really serious. This guy was paying attention to me. I didn't know when to date again. I kept things bottled up. I didn't see a therapist."

When Michael finally left that relationship, he got involved in AIDS activism: "It was a good way for me to release anger I had about AIDS. I felt cheated when Steven died and left me all alone. It was cathartic to yell and scream about AIDS. Being on TV didn't hurt either."

Michael then went on and helped to create a privately funded needle exchange program in Washington, DC, that could be run by community-based groups. The legislation, which Michael helped to write, was passed by Congress in 1996. Through this work, Michael became a local celebrity. He won a few medals, including the "unsung hero" award from Whitman–Walker Clinic, the *Washington Blade* did a story on him, and he was a Grand Marshal in the DC Gay Pride Parade.

Michael saved himself emotionally through activism. He is alone now, but he feels proud of what he's done for the community—a community where "there's no support for being a widower," he said.

Disenfranchised Grief

When your partner dies of AIDS, whether or not you both experienced the Lazarus syndrome, anticipatory grief gives way to bereavement. Unfortunately, the natural process of mourning this loss is often disrupted by the fact that the hurt is not validated by others. Kenneth Doka, a researcher in the field of grief studies, defines this as disenfranchised grief, and says it occurs when one or more of the following occur:

- The relationship is not recognized
- The loss is not recognized
- The griever is not recognized[10]

A classic example of disenfranchised grief is the experience of a mistress versus that of the wife, for whom the latter society creates mechanisms, including fashion (e.g., the black dress), that support and validate the loss. Six weeks prior to my partner's death, my next-door neighbor's husband died. He was a gentle man who often sat on the porch and looked out over our block with a watchful eye. Another neighbor explained to me that a tradition existed on our street, Allison Street, to take up a collection for the family of the deceased and present it to them. I dutifully wrote out a check and also followed up with an orchid plant and visit shortly thereafter. However, my neighbors, who were aware of Jerry's death, since the story was featured on the front pages of *The New York Times* and the *Washington Post,* chose not to follow the Allison Street tradition. Their inaction was symbolic of the very lack of valida-

> **The natural process of mourning is often disrupted by the fact that the hurt is not validated by others.**

tion described above. Though society as a whole does not respond with the same compassion when men experience loss—as in the loss of a wife—my situation was complicated by the fact that we were gay men, one of whom died of AIDS and the other of whom is HIV positive.

While my immediate neighbors responded with inaction, those within my "community of choice" (not unlike the family of choice discussed in Chapter 6), a broad network of friends, family, and coworkers, provided that needed care and support to help me through my grieving process. By my side throughout, whether at his grave site at the family plot in rural Nebraska or at the memorial service at the Metropolitan Community Church (a predominately gay Christian denomination), were Jerry's parents and brother. My experience in that sense was a positive one and contrasts with that of many gay men, who are shut out by their deceased partner's family.

Inge B. Corless, director of the HIV/AIDS Specialization at the Massachusetts General Hospital Institute of Health Professions, recognizes the importance of this kind of support for both partner and parents when she writes, "From another perspective, the family that ostracizes the partner of their son loses a valuable resource for a continuing bond with their son and the man with whom the son has developed a valued relationship. By cutting themselves off from this aspect of their son's development, families lose connection with their son's present life and are restricted to a past of their own making. As ostensibly comforting as this may appear, it reduces the potential sources of support."[11]

Beginning Again: Love after Loss

The linen of shrouds and wedding veils are both made of the same cloth.

—Unknown

On August 15, the first anniversary of Jerry's death, while sailing on the Potomac, I met the next man who would express his love for me. Strangely and perhaps fittingly, he came to the realization of those feelings when he too faced his own mortality—several months later as we lay in the darkness he told me of walking down a dark and unfamiliar city street earlier that night. There he encountered a group of thugs obviously intent on no good. Though he managed to escape unharmed, he realized that if he did indeed die that night it would have been with regret that up till now he had failed to express his love for me.

Though we were together for only a little over a year, he made me understand that it is possible to love again. We spent the time weaving our lives together—traveling, working in my garden, going to concerts together. His was a calming and reassuring presence and one that made me feel safe at a point when I needed it. He also showed me that he could love me independent of my HIV status, and when the relationship ended it happened the way it could have with any other couple, for reasons other than HIV. It also caused me to see another unlikely way in which the risk of loss (in this case nearly losing his life to possible violence) can be a springboard to intimacy. He also came to understand the value of living in the moment. While facing his own mortality, for a brief moment, he saw like many of us with HIV, that joy, love, and happiness are things we are all entitled to and should actively pursue.

Men and Grief

The guidelines and allowance for men to mourn are unclear (see the box on the stages of grief). This is even more true for gay men who mourn the passing of their lovers. Different societies have prescribed periods of mourning—such as sitting shiva in the

THE STAGES OF GRIEF IN ILLNESS AND DEATH

Stage One: Shock

The first stage of grieving is shock. You do not believe the news, and essentially become numb.

Tips and Techniques

When you are in the shock stage and cannot believe the news about the diagnosis or death, you need to:

- Talk to someone about the news and your feelings. The person with the diagnosis and the family should share their feelings with each other if possible and with other family members. It may be helpful to use expert listeners, such as trained clergy, mental health counselors, social workers and nurses. Support groups are wonderful help.
- Be with loved ones who can provide support.
- Hear genuine caring, not suggestions to "fix" the grief. Empathy goes a long way.
- Be encouraged to keep lists of schedules, marked on calendars. It's easy to forget things during this stage of grief. Reminders can be very helpful.

Stage Two: Adjusting

The second stage is the initial adjustment process.

Tips and Techniques

If you are in the second stage of grieving, try the following techniques:

- Realize that what is lost, but remember what remains each day.
- Engage in physical exertion and keep busy to deal with anger or frustration about the situation. Swim laps, go to the gym, take walks, or make bread to help vent intense feelings.
- Get out by yourself and look at peaceful scenes such as a flower garden, go to a museum or spend quiet time at a local church, chapel or synagogue.
- Write down feelings on paper. It helps to keep a diary to review past experiences and gain some perspective. It helps to wad up the paper filled with words and toss it vigorously into the trash, a symbol of throwing away the anger.
- Express yourself in painting or music. *(continued on next page)*

(continued from previous page)

Stage Three: The New Life

In this stage, you take steps to move on to the next phase of your life.

Tips and Techniques

Be encouraged to:

- Seek the company of a pet, a friend or support group if you are feeling lonely or isolated.
- Do something that is different or fun. Indulge in a movie or special treat.
- Be with people. Go to a concert or a free lecture at the public library. Being around happy, healthy people can be healing.
- Try to remember what used to be fun and who used to be fun. Renew former activities and friendships.
- Volunteer. Help others as a way to help yourself. Share what you have learned in your journey with others who are just beginning their journey.

Jewish religion (covering the mirrors and wearing black for seven days) or the nineteenth-century Western European/American tradition of wearing black for a year. For us the most visible symbol for those who died of AIDS has been the Memorial Quilt, which has grown so large and fragile it is unlikely ever to be seen in its entirety again since it was unrolled on the National Mall in Washington in 1996 (see the box on the AIDS Quilt). While the Quilt is a creative and touching memorial to those we've lost, we still may need guidance on how to reenter the world of meeting and dating men again.

Will I Ever Fall in Love Again?

For those of us who have lost a significant other, at some point in our lives the question arises "Will I ever fall in love again?" The accompanying question is "When is the appropriate time to start a new relationship?"

To alleviate the uncertainty and anxiety that can often accompany dating and the process of finding a new relationship, I found it helpful for my clients to manage the process by experiencing it as a sequence of events:

- *Morph and blend.* Recognize that loss is a period of incredible transformation and metamorphosis. Immediately following your loss, you may face an initial period of intense support from people who shared in the life of you and your lover. After a period of time, you may notice that you will interact less and less with people overall, especially with certain people who were closer to your partner than they were with you. This is when you may need more time alone for reflection and the integration of loss, while simultaneously creating a new identity as a single individual.

   However, there will come a time, whether through encouragement from friends or through your own initiative, when you increase your social activities and begin to meet and blend new people into your life.
- *Socialize and date.* As you meet new people, in the course of your day-to-day life or as your hobbies resume after taking a hiatus during your partner's illness, you may meet someone that you *naturally* feel attracted to or vice versa. Recognize

THE AIDS QUILT

In June of 1987, a small group of strangers gathered in a San Francisco storefront to document the lives they feared history would neglect. Their goal was to create a memorial for those who had died of AIDS and thereby to help people understand the devastating impact of the disease. This meeting of devoted friends and lovers served as the foundation of the NAMES Project AIDS Memorial Quilt.

Today the Quilt is a powerful visual reminder of the AIDS pandemic. More than 44,000 individual three-by-six-foot memorial panels—each one commemorating the life of someone who has died of AIDS—have been sewn together by friends, lovers, and family members. The main goal of the Quilt is to provide a creative means for remembrance and healing. For information on how to make a panel and be in the supportive company of others who seek a constructive means to handle their grief, visit their web page at *www.aidsquilt.org*. Local chapters exist across the country.

that these feelings do not invalidate your feelings for your deceased partner but can exist side by side with those feelings. When this occurs, you will know that you are in the right place to date and possibly begin a new relationship again.

> **There will come a time, whether through encouragement from friends or through your own initiative, when you begin to meet and blend new people into your life.**

- *Disclosure.* The delightful and sometimes tricky part about dating is the process of getting to know each other. In that process, you may feel open enough to this new person to reveal that you experienced a recent loss in your life, which may trigger questions about causes of death and your own HIV status. Disclosure, a subject I covered in Chapter 1, needs to be revisited. You may be placed in the paradoxical situation of revealing your HIV-negative status if you happened to be in a serodiscordant relationship.

If and when your new relationship ends, you may find yourself reexperiencing some of the same types of feelings of grief and loss you had after the death of your lover. Remember, you are the keeper of your own heart. Your tenderness may actually serve you and provide an opening to new love, but it needs to be cared for when you face the often inevitable pangs of loss again.

Last Love/New Life: A Sperm Donor, Two Lovers, and Their Child

Do you believe in Life after Love?
—Cher

Mary Grace began thinking about having a child in 1981. It wasn't until four years later that that wish came true. Amelia was born.

As I approached the small house, which was edged in purple and sat on a hill, I looked forward to having Hanukkah dinner with Charlotte, Mary Grace's surviving partner, and Amelia, who at age thirteen would almost be considered a workaholic, with all her extracurricular activities—starring in school plays and being active in sports as well as her school band.

As Amelia's golden hair sparkled next to the menorah candles she lit, she explained, "I'm reading the prayers for all eight nights tonight, as we are going away for Christmas." In the middle of the prayer, Charlotte, with wiry gray hair, yelped out, "Shit," as she burned herself on the fresh potato latkes.

As this was my first Hanukkah dinner, she later explained the importance of timing the expletives just right during the prayer, while giving me a hearty laugh and encouraging me to eat more, in a voice that somehow was both maternal and sounded like an order from a drill sergeant.

After dinner and instructing Amelia to go to her room to finish reading *Don Quixote* for school the next day, she began, "It was 1969 and we were both VISTA volunteers in New Hampshire.

"I was twenty-two, and Mary Grace was nineteen. I had no idea I was queer until she walked into the room and I felt it in my stomach. We were together two years and then broke up, as Mary Grace wasn't really sure if she was gay or not. Over the years we kept in touch—calling on each other's birthdays and writing letters as we began and ended relationships with different people."

Toward the end of a fourteen-year-relationship for Charlotte, she was free to again intensify her affair with Mary Grace.

It was the donated sperm of two gay men—friends of Mary Grace who were involved in a partnered relationship—that succeeded (after twelve attempts) in beginning a new life, as well as eventually ending her own.

Over the years the two women spoke of getting back together again, but they always found a reason or an excuse for it not to happen. It was a phone call in 1989 that knocked away those barriers. "As soon as she told me, I hung up the phone and called Whitman–Walker Clinic," Charlotte continued. "I spoke to one man after another, none of whom could really help me. Finally I asked to speak to the most senior woman of their staff, and she spent two hours on the phone explaining everything to me about HIV, treatment options, and even the importance of safer sex between two women."

Mary Grace, who was described as "poor as a church mouse," was told by Charlotte based on her desperate research that the best medical care was available in either New York City, San Francisco, or here in Washington, DC. A decision was made for Mary Grace to leave Arkansas and for the time being entrust the care of her four-year-old daughter, Amelia, to her former partner and move to be with Charlotte again in Washington: "When I picked her up at the airport, I had decided to start a relationship again, as I had loved her forever and this was a chance to have her back in my life no matter the cost. HIV removed the barriers between us."

Mary Grace was not happy that first month, Charlotte said. "She cried because of the separation from her daughter, and I had a $700 telephone bill that month after she returned." Within a year Amelia, who wanted a house with a "climbing tree," had moved from Arkansas to Washington and back with her mother and Charlotte.

Charlotte stopped her story on occasion to bring up clothes from the dryer to fold, or to yell into the next room to find out what page Amelia was on. "Seventy-two" comes back a tired young voice. Charlotte folds and speaks: "I was angry at those men who went to bathhouses and angry at this fucking disease. Mary Grace called the men who had agreed to donate their sperm and cried angrily to them, 'Do you have something to tell me?!' to which they replied, 'We thought you were all right,' basing this assumption on the good health of Amelia and being unaware of Mary Grace's status."

Amelia later told me she remembered being tested "lots and lots of times, maybe five, but it could have been twenty." Charlotte added, "I put my foot down and told her [Mary Grace] to stop testing her, as she was indeed all right." Now, techniques such as sperm washing, which was first developed in Italy, may allow HIV-positive men to become fathers (although controlled comparative clinical trial data are still needed to support this), while the use of triple-combination therapy with pregnant positive women can also greatly reduce the chance of passing the virus on to an unborn child.

Amelia's biological father died in 1990, and Amelia, who has the cheekbones and coloring of her dad, keeps his picture, as well as Mary Grace's, in her bedroom. Charlotte tells me the two men broke up before his death and believes that "the surviving partner has guilt about that"—a choice that was not an option for these two (reunited by unlikely misfortune) lovers.

Mary Grace began AZT in 1989 and suffered through headaches and fatigue, all the while insisting on working. "When Mary Grace was sick, she was the opposite of me and would go into her room and when approached would yell, 'Leave me alone—the hell alone,'" Charlotte said. During this time, not much was known about the unique treatment needs of women with HIV. In fact, research and treatment for women even lags behind that which is available for men today.

Complications from AIDS

Mary Grace eventually joined a support group for women with HIV and developed close bonds, which Charlotte still maintains with the one surviving woman. One member, a mutual friend of ours, died of what was called "complications from AIDS" in her obituary, which involved putting a bullet in her own head, partly because she did not want to go through this disease alone.

Complications soon became apparent in Mary Grace's life. As she became more tired, she decided to retire from her job at a nonprofit organization and spend more time raising her daughter, "puttering around the house, working on her arts and crafts, as well as the garden." Mary Grace was open to alternative medicine and received massages and did Chinese medicine. "I would snicker, but that was OK," Charlotte shared.

March 1995 saw the first time she was in the hospital with a "horrible ulcer on her throat," requiring her to be put on a liquid diet, which resulted in a loss of thirty pounds in two weeks, going from 145 to 115.

Charlotte struggled to put together the memories of that period: "Time changes for me. . . . It blends into itself because it was something horrible." Not clearly remembering the second of a series of trips to the hospital, she goes on: "The third time she complained of a pain in her side, and Amelia saw a growth pop up on her neck. Mary Grace would need surgery and need to be placed on a lung pump. Recalling the sound of that machine, which she was on for thirty days, made us decide not to put a water garden in." What is normally considered the peaceful sound of water gurgling is now forever imprinted with her partner's suffering: "I spent every night with her in the hospital, came home and fed Amelia breakfast, and then went to work."

During that time and after, their daughter has provided Charlotte with a reason to cope: "Had I not had Amelia to take care of, I would still be unable to live and function. Because she [Amelia] had to live. I had this kid who had to have three meals a day, do homework, and try to have fun."

For women who are the partners and primary caretakers of those who progress in illness, their increase in responsibility is not often met with an increase in support services. As the face of HIV becomes more feminine, increasing service delivery from double-duty clinics like the one at Georgetown Hospital's Infectious Disease Program that offers pediatric care while the mothers are receiving treatment for their HIV will need to become more familiar models of care.

Amelia, at the time of our interview, was a young girl with tremendous life energy, had played the lead role in her school play, was learning the violin, and was active in her school's wrestling team. Also, as is often the case with those with so much energy, especially during the teenage years, she was "grounded not for life, but until she straightens up her act a bit more."

During the final weeks of her life, Mary Grace suffered from dementia and believed that "the waffle iron was chirping at her." Charlotte recalls the anger when she told Mary Grace she couldn't drive anymore due to her detached retinas from the CMV. As she shared that, I recalled a phone call I received from a DC taxi driver with whom my partner had had a fender bender due to his own progressive illness, and my having to insist he give up his license as well.

As was stated before, the process of grief begins before the actual loss of a loved one, but people experience these losses with different abilities and levels of independence. "I had never felt so hopeless. . . . To see someone so vibrant, intelligent and alive gradually change to being like a child of three or four," Charlotte said. Through the tears she adds, "I feel angry because her cognitive abilities were gone and I couldn't say good-bye." Turning to me she said, "I don 't know what it is like for a man, but the moment they put a tube in her breast—that she had breast-fed Amelia with—she stopped feeling like a woman."

In a follow-up interview, Amelia shared with me her own memories of her mother: "I remember little funny things. . . . Us laughing in the car because my Mom had to go to the bathroom and I told her to think of 'something nonliquid like a stone' and she said, 'My pee is as heavy as a stone.' "

Closure was accomplished between mother and child when, during a moment of clarity during her last week alive in the hospital, she told her, "Mia, I love you." This is believed to have been one of Mary Grace's last verbal communications.

Surrounded by friends and Charlotte, Mary Grace, at 5:30 A.M., opened her eyes and said clearly, "God," as she sat up in bed. "Then, I knew, the doors had opened for her," Charlotte said. "Earlier I had crawled in the hospital bed with her as she was tossing and turning, and she calmed down and slept in my arms.

"Later while sitting next to her and holding her hand I told her it was all right and to go where she had to go. The nurses came in and all said good-bye and later talked about what a peaceful death she had."

During that time, "I was struck by the goodness of people to Amelia and me. I remember coming home that night and crying because it had been weeks since Mary Grace and I had slept in our bed together. For weeks afterward I took her picture to bed with me, and it still is the last thing I see when I go to bed at night and the first thing I see when I awake in the morning."

Mary Grace's artwork hangs on the wall. Her daughter reports she is on page seventy-six of her reading assignment. I share with Charlotte my feeling that the "homework of loss" continues and that having been present at the last moments of our loved ones' lives and providing comfort to them helps us to complete that ongoing homework.

Charlotte and Mary Grace shared the youthful process of self-discovery and the much-hoped-for experience of first love. As years and other relationships passed, their relationship also became the realization of a different, unsung, less-written-about "last love."

AIDS, like adolescence, is a time of profound change, both physically and emotionally, and relationships against these backdrops are imbued with a unique intensity and passion. We will always remember our first loves for that reason; and for the same reasons, we will always cherish the memory of being someone's last love.

EPILOGUE

The role of a good therapist or reporter is to be a biographer or chronicler of people's lives, often bringing a bit of objectiveness and clarity to what is sometimes a painful subject.

Recognizing I may not be able to do that about my own life or the one I shared with my former partner Jerry, I offer the following from Paula Span (*Washington Post Magazine*, copyright 2001):

> Still would he have met the love of his life if he hadn't been HIV Positive? . . . At a financial planning workshop for people with HIV he met a pale Midwestern lawyer who worked at the Justice Department. "If he hadn't been ill," Mancilla says, "he probably would've been the first gay senator from Nebraska."
>
> Jerry Roemer's presence is still everywhere in the art-filled row house they bought together. The portrait taken at their 1995 commitment ceremony is prominent among the clutter of family photos on the mantle: Roemer wore a tux: Mancilla sported a dinner jacket ("I always wanted to wear white"); they jointly clutched a spray of orchids and lilies.

Based on both my personal and professional life, it remains my firm belief that the possibilities for love while living with HIV are greater now than ever before. I hope this book helped you to begin to believe this as well.

Love becomes greater and nobler in calamity.
—Gabriel Garciá Márquez,
Love in the Time of Cholera

APPENDIX A

LEGAL PROTECTIONS FOR COUPLES WITH HIV

LIZ SEATON[1]

This is a general guide to legal protections for people with HIV. It is not legal advice and should not be taken or followed as such. I hope to highlight some important decision-making issues—health care, financial planning, property rights, and family law—that you may want to deal with proactively when one or both people in a couple relationship are HIV positive.

Most of the laws addressing these various issues are state laws, meaning that they differ from state to state, although a few federal laws also come into play. You probably want to become familiar with the law in your state, but keep in mind that law is full of nuances and technicalities. I would be remiss if I did not tell you that there is simply no substitute for legal advice specific to the law in your state, tailored to your own situation, and provided by a good lawyer. I encourage you to seek counsel.

How Do You Find a Lawyer When You Need One?

Many areas around the country have legal services programs tailored to meet the legal needs of people living with HIV, though to qualify for some you must meet stringent low-income and asset guidelines. Ask an HIV service provider to refer you to a legal services program in your area, or at least in your state. Even if you are not eligible to be represented by one of their lawyers, they may have a referral list of private attorneys who have expressed an interest in representing people with HIV, and they probably have some form documents that you could use. The American Bar Association's HIV/AIDS Coordination Project has a *Directory of Legal Resources for People with AIDS and HIV* (published in Washington, DC) that could help you to locate an HIV legal service provider in your area.

If you find that you need to hire a private attorney, try to work with one that you know something about and with whom you feel comfortable. Ask your family and friends to refer you to a lawyer who did a good job for them, or maybe someone in your support group knows an attorney. Also, get in touch with your state and local bar associations. Often they operate a lawyer referral service.

Remember that lawyers tend to specialize in just a few areas, so you may want to question your potential lawyer about his or her training and/ or experience in the area with which you need help. It is worth noting that a lawyer who is not an expert in your topic of law but works diligently for you and is willing to seek out expert advice as necessary may be more valuable than an expert in the field who is too busy to really give your issues and questions full attention.

Be Proactive in Communicating with Your Lawyer

Keep in mind that what seems obvious to you may not be to your lawyer. To get things clear in your own mind, write down what you hope to accomplish and any questions that you have before meeting with the lawyer. The more openly and honestly you communicate about your situation, the more likely you are to get the best advice and product from your lawyer.

What seems obvious to your lawyer undoubtedly will not be to you. For example, for reasons relating to protecting the person's wishes and confidentiality, an attorney may want to meet with a person alone rather than with his partner, at least for the initial visit. Remember that the law has its limits in terms of what kinds of arrangements a person can make, though a creative lawyer can sometimes figure out ways to expand the available options. Lawyers also have a way of talking in attorney shorthand.

Don't be shy; keep asking questions until you understand exactly what the lawyer is saying and know all of your options.

Finally, it helps to clarify the fee arrangement in advance and in writing. If you are seeing a legal services attorney, you should ask: Is the work being performed pro bono (for free)? Or will you be charged a sliding scale fee (based on their rules about how much you have to pay depending on how much income you have)? If you are seeing a private attorney, will there be a flat fee, or does the lawyer charge by the hour, and, if so, how many hours does she anticipate working on your case? Ask any lawyer you visit if you will need to pay other costs such as filing fees (fees charged by a court or agency to hear your case).

Marriage Provides the Most Protection for Couples: What Can We Do?

Though many people have questions about the value of the institution of marriage, it offers the most comprehensive package of legal protections to a couple. Marriage confers more than a thousand federal and hundreds of state rights and benefits. These can be shared benefits like health insurance, pensions, and Social Security; family rights such as presumption of paternity (fatherhood) and strong parental rights; next-of-kin powers such as decision-making authority and the right to inherit; and more. (Marriage also gives partners a set of obligations to one another, most notable of which are fidelity and a level of basic support including food, housing, and clothing, and, in some states, medical care.)

Heterosexual couples can marry in every country in the world. Unfortunately, only same-sex couples who are nationals of the Netherlands (since 2001) and Belgium (2003) enjoy the right to marry. Canada seems poised to enact same-sex marriage, with both the Canadian Parliament and the Canadian Supreme Court under pressure since two lower courts ruled that keeping same-sex couples from marriage violates the Canadian Charter of Rights and Freedoms. As of this writing, only one U.S. state, Vermont, has enacted legislation that duplicates the state-level (but not federal) benefits of marriage for same-sex couples who enter into a "civil union." Over the past few years, in anticipation of same-sex couples traveling to whatever becomes the first state to enact full same-sex marriage and then returning home with marriage certificates, thirty-six states (Alabama, Alaska, Arizona, Arkansas, California, Colorado, Delaware, Florida, Georgia, Hawaii, Idaho, Illinois, Indiana, Iowa, Kansas, Kentucky, Louisiana, Maine, Michigan, Minnesota, Mississippi, Missouri, Montana, Nebraska, North Carolina, North Dakota, Oklahoma, Pennsylvania, South Carolina, South Dakota, Tennessee, Texas, Utah, Virginia, Washington, and West Virginia) have passed laws banning the recognition of same-sex marriages within their borders. In states where these specific bans have not been enacted, no same-sex marriages have been performed. Also, it is unclear whether same-sex marriages performed someday in another state will be honored.

Several countries, including Denmark, Finland, France, Germany, Iceland, Norway, and Sweden, have broad domestic partnership laws that offer a significant package of rights. Also, in a few states (California, Connecticut, and Hawaii) and some U.S. cities, unmarried couples are permitted to register as domestic partners, with typically a very limited set of between one and ten rights and benefits attached to the partnership. San Francisco and New York City have the most comprehensive local domestic partnership laws in the country. Though many people feel that domestic partnership is a good alternative to marriage, none of the U.S. state laws or city ordinances establishing domestic partnerships confer anywhere near the comprehensive package of benefits on a couple that marriage does. (Some companies offer benefits to their employees' domestic partners; check with your workplace's personnel office.)

For these reasons, effective personal planning for unmarried couples, whether HIV positive or not, frequently involves preparing papers and having them properly signed, witnessed, and even notarized. It is important to leave your documents in safe hands with someone who will know if something happens to you, since that person will need to actively step forward with them at the appropriate moment.

Because the focus of this book is on dating and forming couples, I give a little information about the law and sexuality. Then I focus on the actions people might take to protect their couple relationships, but it also is wise to consider what may happen if the relationship ends. If two people marry, they will also be subject to state laws dealing with dividing property and settling any disputes over the custody of children if they divorce. State laws have also sometimes been applied to same-sex breakups, but this is also an area where courts in several states have balked and refused to deal with these cases at all. Some couples, in a proactive move to help ease the conflict in the event the relationship ends, put into writing "partnership agreements"—their plans for splitting up the money and property in the event that they split up. Many courts are enforcing these types of contracts, but again this is an issue that differs by jurisdiction.

Some States Still Criminalize Consensual Adult Relationships

Alabama, Florida, Idaho, Kansas, Louisiana, Missouri, Mississippi, North Carolina, Oklahoma, South Carolina, Texas, Utah, and Virginia: these thirteen states still have some form of a criminal sodomy law (not specific to HIV/AIDS, but alarming nonetheless) on the books in an enforceable way. This means that you can be arrested, convicted, fined and even sentenced to prison for engaging in the sexual acts—usually defined as oral and/or anal sex—that the state deems illegal. As a practical matter, these laws are often not enforced; if they *are* enforced, they are often applied to people engaging in public sex. It perhaps does not need to be said that most often these laws are used to prosecute gay men in "sting" operations. However, in an important case now pending before the U.S. Supreme Court called *Lawrence v. State,* two men in Texas were convicted for having sex in the privacy of one of their homes. It is also worth noting that while Michigan's sodomy law was ruled unconstitutional, the state prosecutes same-sex sexual conduct under the "indecency and immorality" statute.

Having HIV Can Raise the Stakes, in Both Criminal and Civil Law

Because HIV is relatively new on the scene in the course of human history, the law is still developing as to how our society addresses and deals with HIV. I think that you should be aware of a few potential problem areas. First, depending on where you live, it can be a crime for a person who is living with HIV to engage in sexual relations with another person. Each state has generic criminal laws that could be used against a person who exposes another person to HIV. As of this writing twenty-seven states have a law criminalizing the transmission of (or even just exposure to) HIV: Arkansas, California, Colorado, Florida, Georgia, Idaho, Illinois, Indiana, Iowa, Kentucky, Louisiana, Maryland, Michigan, Missouri, Nevada, New Jersey, North Dakota, Ohio, Oklahoma, Pennsylvania, South Carolina,

South Dakota, Tennessee, Vermont, Virginia, Washington, and Wisconsin. Second, in some states people have won civil lawsuits against a former sexual partner with HIV for exposing them to the virus. The safer course of action legally speaking is to engage only in protected or safe sex with a partner to whom you can prove that you disclosed your HIV status and from whom you got affirmative consent.

Making Sure Your Health Care Providers Know What Care You Want

If you are conscious (and not mentally incapacitated), you can talk with your doctor about your own wishes about your health care and act as your own advocate. For some reason that is not entirely clear to me, people worry that if they write down their wishes in a legal document (see below), their doctor will read the piece of paper and follow its instructions rather than talking with them about their medical options. I encourage you to write your wishes down. Most doctors want to maintain good relationships with their patients (and avoid lawsuits) and will communicate with them directly if at all possible.

No matter how healthy or ill you are, you may want to express your wishes regarding health care in a document called a *living will*. You specify your wishes in writing (e.g., that you want pain medication to keep you comfortable or that you do not want your heart restarted if it stops). What goes into this document is personal to you, and you should think carefully about it. It will be used in the event that you cannot communicate. (Please be aware that this document will not guarantee that you will get health care; all it means is that a doctor providing you with health care must pay attention to your wishes.)

Remember, Keep Your Private Health Insurance to Give You the Most Options

It almost never pays to give up private health insurance, thinking that you can use a publicly funded program such as AIDS drug assistance programs, Medicaid, or Medicare (and, by the way, Medicare does not yet cover prescription drugs). First, most public programs have pretty stringent limitations on income and assets to qualify. Second, usually the coverage is not as comprehensive as that of private health insurance, and they tend to give you far fewer options about where you receive health care. Third, you never know when the government might decide to change its programs or its eligibility criteria—especially with most states facing significant budget shortfalls as of 2003.

Naming Your Partner to Make Decisions for You If You Can't Do So

It is impossible for a person to write down, in advance, his wishes for every possible medical situation that might arise. You might need a trusted person, perhaps your partner, to act as your advocate in a health care setting. In every state, the law says that the legal next of kin, a spouse if there is one, then children if they are grown, etc., have the right to make decisions for someone who is incapacitated.

To get around that rule, you can use a document often called a *health care power of attorney*. In it, you name the person to make health care decisions not addressed in the person's living will. It makes sense to choose a person to act as health care power of attorney who has agreed to advocate for the kind of health care the person who signs over the authority actually wants. In other words, talk about your wishes very specifically, and be sure that whoever you name understands your wishes and agrees to comply with them.

Each state's rules are different, so you want to get the form that works for your state (ask an HIV service provider or local hospital to provide you with one). Most doctors in other states will honor a health care power of attorney form from another state, but if you travel regularly to one other state, you may want to get that state's form too.

The rules vary by state, but all of these documents need to be signed in front of qualified witnesses, and sometimes they must be notarized. Often banks offer notary services, and notaries are listed in the phone book.

The beauty of the health care power of attorney form is that it helps a partner who is otherwise legally unrelated to gain access to the doctor's office and/or hospital room. In addition, in most areas where domestic partnership exists because of state or local laws, the partners are guaranteed access to each other in health care settings. Obviously married couples are permitted access, and generally so are other legal family members.

Arrange for Someone
to Take Care of Your Finances If You Can't Do So

Lots of couples arrange for the future care of their individual finances by commingling their money in shared accounts and in joint ownership of personal property (e.g., checking accounts or cars) and real property (land and buildings). People do this by signing documents as joint tenants with right of survivorship or tenants in common—ask an attorney to explain the differences to you, because they are important. While this does offer flexibility because each person can then deal with many different types of financial transactions, it makes sense to enter these types of arrangements by considering the short- and long-term consequences in view of anticipated illness or death. There may be other important questions to ask if one or both of you have HIV, but at least two that come to mind: First, what will happen to the jointly held money or property if one person goes deeply into debt to pay for expensive prescription drugs and medical care? Second, does commingling the finances disqualify one partner for public benefits—especially Social Security, Medicaid, or HIV/AIDS Drug Assistance—to which he might otherwise be entitled?

To name someone else to take care of finances, in all states you can complete a form called a *durable power of attorney*. The powers granted to the person with the power of attorney are those written into the document, so they can be very broad or very limited. Depending on the form and the laws of the state, the powers given in the document can either start immediately or spring into effect when the person becomes incapacitated; the form probably has to be notarized. Basically the way this form works is that the person named as the power of attorney takes the form to conduct business on the other person's behalf. Remember that the person holding the power of attorney needs to specify that he or she is signing *with the power of attorney for the other person*. To do this, the person with the power of attorney simply signs his name as usual, then writes *POA* after it. Especially be careful at the hospital; if you sign just your name when your partner is admitted without specifying your power of attorney, you might well end up ultimately being responsible for paying for his expensive medical bills.

Three other special financial situations come to mind: First, the Social Security Administration does not recognize these forms; it has a different mechanism called "representative payee" for situations where one person is handling Social Security benefits for another. Second, many banks would rather have whoever is named as a durable power of attorney fill out a card-sized form that fits neatly into the bank's signature card box. Finally, even a person named as durable power of attorney cannot sign a last will and testament for another person.

Among the less commonly used financial planning tools are *inter vivos* trusts (naming an original trustee and a successor trustee), which are expensive to maintain and most useful for wealthy people and conservatorships (sometimes called *guardianships;* they usually require a court proceeding and deprive the "ward" of autonomy and self-determination).

Dealing with Property Rights in Case You Die

When you die, your property goes to your legal next of kin, unless other arrangements have been made. This cannot be emphasized too strongly: if each person in an unmarried couple wants his partner to have his assets, the couple must make specific arrangements and follow all of the rules very carefully. I have all too often encountered couples that erroneously believed that because they lived together they were each other's legal heirs, only to be devastated to discover they were wrong when the legal spouse or biological family arrived and asserted their rights. At the risk of sounding too mercenary, it pays a couple to be proactive.

In cases where a couple can predict with some certainty that one partner will likely die in the near future, you may want to meet with a lawyer to discuss options for protecting the couple's assets. Obviously this can be a very emotional time, but it may be worth it to the couple to explore two things: First, whether the couple's property is set up so that the surviving partner will have enough cash immediately available to deal with burial/cremation, pay for any religious services, and also continue to meet his daily living expenses. Second, it is possible that some inheritance taxes could be avoided if one partner, while still living, transfers property to his anticipated surviving partner.

Once a person dies, the state legal processes for dealing with most of the deceased partner's money, property, debts, etc., are called *probate procedures,* and they are carried out in *probate courts.* (It is also worth noting that any power of attorney forms that were in effect while the person was alive are now useless.) Some property may transfer to another person automatically (we lawyers call this "by operation of law") without having to go through the probate procedures, for example where finances are commingled. The title to bank accounts and personal and real property can all be set up to transfer automatically to another person when someone dies, though there are very specific rules for making these arrangements. A person can name his partner to be the beneficiary of his life insurance policy, though in some states even if a gay partner still has a legal spouse, she has some rights related to life insurance. Typically this means that a spouse who will not be a beneficiary must give written permission for someone else to be the beneficiary.

To make probate work seamlessly for an unmarried couple, each person must have a last will and testament that names the other partner as his *beneficiary*—in other words, the person to whom he leaves his belongings. In some states, there is a mandatory percentage that must be left to a legal spouse, if one exists. In case a family member decides to challenge a will, it is extremely important to have followed all of the rules about signing, witnessing, and notarizing the will. For the will to work, it must be filed with the probate court in the county where the person most recently resided quite soon after the person dies.

Making Plans in Advance for the Custody of Your Children, Just in Case

This can be a complex area of the law; see an attorney to make arrangements for the future care of children, including formalizing an already existing arrangement (e.g., your unmarried partner really serves as your child's other parent). In the area of family law, HIV legal service providers often can help only with arrangements where everyone agrees who will be the future caregivers. Don't hesitate to ask whether your lawyer knows of other organizations or bar association programs that can provide low- or no-cost services to families with low incomes.

The options for naming the future caregiver of children vary widely from state to state. Biological parents have extremely strong parental rights: if one parent dies and the second biological parent is known, still living, and his or her parental rights have not been terminated, he or she may have the right to take custody regardless of whether he or she has been significantly involved in caregiving to date. If there are two known biological parents, both of whom are still living, it greatly simplifies future care arrangements if both parents can agree and cooperate in setting it up.

With that in mind, let me list a few types of arrangements for the future care of children, keeping in mind that there may be more or less options available in any given state:

1. *Testamentary guardianship*—a parent can use a last will and testament to nominate a person to become the legal custodian of his or her children after his or her death (but the court that reads the will still has the power to approve or disapprove the nomination).
2. *Custody or adoption hearing*—some parents, seeking the peace of mind that comes with certainty, give up parental rights to a child and allow the future caregiver to take custody in a consent proceeding during the parent's lifetime. A few states allow a parent and an anticipated future caregiver to take joint custody of children, which means that the parent retains her rights up until death and then the new legal caregiver is already in place.
3. *Springing guardianship*—some states allow a parent to fill out papers that will spring into effect if she dies, putting in place the parent's choice of a legal guardian for her children, although often these types of arrangements are for a specific, limited period of time. Once the papers expire, the family will need to go to court to make the arrangement permanent.

What If You Know What You Want Done with Your Body When You Die?

Many people (at least in the industrialized countries) are living with HIV these days, not dying from it, but since there is little information about this subject, I feel compelled to include it. If you know exactly what you want done with your body, some states will permit you to make a burial directive, specifying the arrangements to be made. This can become a little complicated, because funeral homes are extremely reluctant to make arrangements without contacting next of kin, even when presented with a proper burial directive. Though this sounds a little grim, it helps to contract with the funeral home to make the arrangements before death if possible. Often it helps to talk with relatives about your wishes about what should happen to your body before you even become ill.

What Else Do You Need to Know?

The law affects all of our daily lives, often in unseen ways. You could have a legal issue arising from your HIV status that is completely unrelated to anything I have discussed here. In employment, insurance, and immigration law, among many other legal areas, HIV plays a significant, complex role. You may have rights of which you are unaware (e.g., protection from HIV discrimination on the job), or your rights may be limited because you have HIV (e.g., in immigration or international travel). We have come full circle now, because I leave you with one of the first pieces of advice I started with: if you have a question about how the law applies to your specific situation, do seek legal counsel.

APPENDIX B

RESOURCES

United States Hotlines

**The Americans with Disabilities Act Information
and Assistance Hotline**
800-514-0301 V/TTY

**The Centers for Disease Control and Prevention (CDC) National
AIDS Clearinghouse (Information and publication orders)**
800-458-5231 (Monday–Friday 9 A.M. to 6 P.M.)

The Gay and Lesbian National Hotline
888-THE-GLNH (888-843-4564) Monday–Friday 6 P.M. to 10 P.M.; Saturday
   12 P.M. to 5 P.M. (Eastern Standard Time)
   This is a nonprofit organization that provides nationwide toll-free peer
counseling, information, and referrals.

Hemophilia AIDS Network/National Hemophilia Foundation
800-424-2634

Helping Individual Prostitutes Survive Hotline
800-676-4477
   For adolescent prostitutes.

National AIDS Hotline
800-342-2437 (24 hours a day, daily)
TTY/TDD: 800-243-7889
English Hotline: 800-342-AIDS
Spanish Hotline: 800-344-SIDA

National Association of People with AIDS
202-898-0414 Hotline and TTY/TDD

National Domestic Violence Hotline
800-799-7233

National Gay and Lesbian Youth Hotline
800-347-TEEN

National Herpes Hotline
919-361-8488

National Prevention Information Network
800-458-5231 (English and Spanish)
TTY/TDD: 800-243-7012
International line: 301-562-1098

A service to get free educational materials about HIV, tuberculosis, and sexually transmitted diseases (STDs).

National Sexually Transmitted Diseases (STD) Hotline
English: 800-227-8922
Spanish: 800-344-7432
TTY/TDD: 800-243-7889

Provides anonymous, confidential information on sexually transmitted diseases (STDs) and how to prevent them. Also, provides referrals to clinical and other services. Open Monday–Friday 8 A.M. to 11 P.M. (Eastern Standard Time).

Rape Abuse and Incest National Network
800-656-HOPE

Treatment Hotlines

AIDS Treatment Data Network
212-260-8868 (local New York City)
Hotline hours: Monday–Friday, 9 A.M. to 5 P. M. (Eastern Standard Time)

Project Inform
National HIV treatment line: 800-822-7422
International Hotline: 415-558-9051
Hotline hours: Monday–Friday: 9 A.M. to 5 P.M.; Saturday: 10 A.M. to 4 P.M. (Pacific Time)

National Clinician's Post-Exposure Prophylaxis Hotline (PEPline)
888-448-4911

National Clinical Trials Hotline
800-TRIALS-A (800-874-2572)
International: 301-519-0459

Callers can speak with experienced health specialists for help in locating HIV/AIDS clinical trials across the United States. Spanish-speaking specialists available.

Pride Institute
800-54-PRIDE

Provides specialized treatment for gays and lesbians in a safe and affirming environment for issues related to HIV/AIDS, substance abuse, depression, and other psychiatric problems. Locations across the United States.

Help for Addiction

Al-Anon (and **Alateen** for younger members)
888-425-2666, in Canada and the United States

A worldwide organization that offers a self-help recovery program for families and friends of alcoholics whether or not the alcoholic seeks help or even recognizes the existence of a drinking problem.

Cocaine Anonymous
National referral line: 800-482-0983

This number is a referral service for updated information only.

Sexual Compulsives Anonymous
800-977-HEAL

Website Directory of National AIDS Organizations

AIDS Action Committee	*www.aac.org*
AIDS Action Council	*www.aidsaction.org*
AIDS Clinical Trials Information Services	*www.actis.org*
AIDS Research Alliance	*www.aidsresearch.org*
AIDS Research Information	*www.critpath.org*

AIDS Treatment Data Network	*www.aidsnyc.org*
AIDS Treatment News	*www.thebody.com*
American Foundation for AIDS Research (AmFAR)	*www.amfar.org*
Centers for Disease Control	*www.cdc.gov*
HIV Information	*www.aegis.com*
International Association of Physicians in AIDS Care	*www.iapac.org*
National Association of People with AIDS	*www.napwa.org*
National Institute of Allergy and Infectious Disease	*www.niaid.nih.gov*
Project Inform	*www.projinf.org*
The Names Project	*www.aidsquilt.org*
Veterans Affairs, HIV Information	*vhaaidsinfo.cio.med.va.gov*
World Health Organization	*www.who.org*

NOTES

Chapter 1

1. George Chauncey, *Gay New York: Gender, Urban Culture, and the Making of the Gay Male World 1890–1940* (New York: Basic Books, 1995).
2. D. Binson et al., "Prevalence and Social Distribution of Men Who Have Sex with Men: United States and Its Social Distribution of Men Who Have Sex with Men—United States and Its Urban Centers," *Journal of Sex Research, 32*(3), 245–254, 1995.
3. Peter G. Keogh & Susan Beardsell, "Sexual Health of HIV-Positive Gay Men," paper presented at the Eleventh International Conference on AIDS, Vancouver, British Columbia, Canada, July 1996.
4. Ibid.
5. Daniel Schnell et al., "Men's Disclosure of HIV Test Results to Primary Male Sex Partners," *American Journal of Public Health, 82,* 1675, 1992.
6. David Nimmons, *The Soul Beneath the Skin: The Unseen Hearts and Habits of Gay Men* (New York: St. Martin's Press, 2002), p. 66.

Chapter 2

1. Susan Sontag, *AIDS and Its Metaphors* (New York: Farrar, Straus & Giroux, 1988), pp. 24–25.
2. David Mann, *Psychotherapy: An Erotic Relationship–Transference and Countertransference Passions* (London: Routledge, 1997).
3. Sheppard B. Kominars & Kathryn D. Kominars, *Accepting Ourselves and Others: A Journey into Recovery from Addictive and Compulsive Behaviors for Gays, Lesbians & Bisexuals* (Center City, MN: Hazelden Press, 1996).

4. Gina Corea, *The Invisible Epidemic: The Story of Women and AIDS* (New York: HarperCollins, 1992).
5. Sally Zierler, Lisa Feingold, et al., "Adult Survivors of Childhood Sexual Abuse and Subsequent Risk of HIV Infection," *American Journal of Public Health, 81*(5), 572–575, 1991.
6. Corea, op. cit., p. 69.
7. Mike Lew, *Victims No Longer: Men Recovering from Incest and other Sexual Child Abuse* (New York: HarperCollins, 1990).
8. L. S. Doll, Joy D. Bartholow et al., "Self-Reported Childhood and Adolescent Sexual Abuse Among Adult Homosexual and Bisexual Men," *Child Abuse and Neglect, 16*, 855–864, 1992.
9. Lew, op. cit., p. xviii.
10. Scott O'Hara, in Dangerous Bedfellows, Wayne Hoffman, & Eva Pendleton (Eds.), *Policing Public Sex: Queer Politics and the Future of AIDS Activism* (Boston: South End Press, 1996), p. 83.

Chapter 3

1. These statements about relative risk were up to date as of the time of publication, but they are constantly being reviewed and may change.
2. Dr. Bruni has changed the location of the patient and other potentially identifying characteristics to protect his confidentiality.
3. Quoted in Rajesh T. Gandi, "Highlights from IDSA: HIV in Genital Secretions," *The Hopkins HIV Report,* January 1999.
4. Troy P. Suarez et al., "Influence of a Partner's Serostatus, Use Of Highly Active Antiretroviral Therapy, and Viral Load on Perceptions of Sexual Risk Behavior in a Community Sample of Men Who Have Sex with Men," *Journal of Acquired Immune Deficiency Syndromes, 28*, 471–477, 2001.
5. It's also worth noting that "undetectable" is a moving target anyway, with the number having shifted over the years. In fact, at one time a patient with a viral load consistently of 250 was deemed suppressed. So, the word *undetectable* should never be assumed to equate with a specific number. What is considered undetectable now may not be tomorrow.

Chapter 4

1. Renee Lyons et al., *Relationships in Chronic Illness and Disability* (Thousand Oaks, CA: Sage, 1995).
2. S. Planalp & K. Garvin-Doxas, in Steven Duck (Ed.), *Dynamics of Relationships* (Thousand Oaks, CA: Sage, 1994), pp. 1–26.

3. J. K. Kiecolt-Glaser et al., "Psychosocial Enhancement of Immunocompetence in a Geriatric Population," *Health Psychology, 4* 25–41, 1985..

4. Lyons et al., op. cit., p. 13.

5. Geoffrey Cowley et al., "Attention Aging Men," *Newsweek, 16,* 73, September 1996.

6. Steven Schwartzberg, *A Crisis of Meaning: How Gay Men Are Making Sense of AIDS* (New York: Oxford University Press, 1996), p. 152.

7. Ibid., p. 150.

8. Lyons et al., op. cit., p.73.

9. Schwartzberg, op. cit., p.64.

10. Lyons et al., op. cit., p.64.

11. Michael Scarce, "The Boys Who Bareback: Ride on the Wild Side," *POZ,* p. 54, February 1999.

12. Drew J. Cohen & Anthony S. Fauci, "Transmission of Multidrug-Resistant HIV: The Wake-up Call," Editorial, *New England Journal of Medicine 339*(5), July 30, 1998.

13. "Survey Shows Increase in Unprotected Sex," *Bay Area Reporter 16,* April 1998.

14. Jesse Green, "Flirting with Suicide: Public Health Campaigns Shout 'Just Say No,' but People Don't Listen. If They Did, Why Would Someone Like Mark Ebenhoch Still Be Having Unsafe Sex?" *New York Times Magazine,* p. 39, September 15, 1996.

15. Bill Strubbe, "Positive and Unprotected," *SF Weekly,* July 9, 1997.

16. Scarce, op. cit., p. 70.

17. Strubbe, op. cit., p. 4.

18. Henry Louis Gates, *Thirteen Ways at Looking at a Black Man* (Hopkinton, MA: Vintage Books, 1998).

Chapter 5

1. I am an assistant professor of law at The John Marshall Law School, Chicago. I wrote this chapter to fulfill a promise made to Jerry Roemer, who was my roommate in Nebraska before I moved to New York and before he moved to Washington, DC, where he met Michael Mancilla, one of the authors of this book. The process of writing this chapter has been emotionally difficult for both of us because of Jerry's untimely death. The protease inhibitors that saved so many others could not save him. I dedicate this chapter to the fond memory of Jerry's love for Michael and Michael's love for Jerry.

2. Mark E. Wojcik, "Prohibiting AIDS Discrimination by Funeral Homes," paper presented at the Tenth International Conference on AIDS, Yokohama, Japan, Abstract 210D, August 7–12, 1994.

3. Personals, *New York Blade*, p. 34, December 4, 1998.

4. Personals, *Washington Blade*, p. 84, December 11, 1998.

5. Ibid., p. 85.

6. Ibid., p. 84.

7. In *Dry Bones Breathe*, Eric Rofes observes that researchers studying HIV-negative men "may be interested in learning how their sexual practices kept them from becoming infected or what kinds of genes they carry that may have kept HIV from taking hold in their systems, but rarely have researchers investigated the social, cultural, and psychological experiences of uninfected men during the epidemic." Eric Rofes, *Dry Bones Breathe: Gay Men Create Post-AIDS Identities and Cultures* Binghamton, NY: Harrington Park Press, 1998), pp. 82–83.

8. Jesse Green, "Flirting with Suicide: Public Health Campaigns Shout 'Just Say No,' but People Don't Listen. If They Did, Why Would Someone Like Mark Ebenhoch Still Be Having Unsafe Sex?" *New York Times Magazine*, p. 39, September 15, 1996.

9. Mark Sullivan, "Study Finds Drop in HIV Infections: Percentage of Gay Men Infected With HIV Plunges by Two-Thirds from a Decade Ago," *New York Blade*, p. 1, December 4, 1998.

10. Walt Odets, *In the Shadow of the Epidemic: Being HIV-Negative in the Age of AIDS* (Durham, NC: Duke University Press, 1995).

11. William I. Johnston, *HIV-Negative: How the Uninfected Are Affected by AIDS* (New York: Insight Books, 1995).

12. Odets, op. cit., p. 17.

13. Johnston, op. cit., p. 96.

14. Ibid., p. 97.

15. Ibid.

16. Odets, op. cit., p. 106.

17. Ibid.

18. Johnston, op. cit., p. 122.

19. Ibid., p. 123.

20. Mark E. Wojcik, "AIDS: What Funeral Directors Need to Know," *John Marshall Law Review*, 27, 411, 1994.

21. Personals, *Washington Blade*, p. 84, December 11, 1998.

22. Johnston, op. cit., p. 170.

23. Ibid., p. 171.

24. Ibid., pp. 171–72.

25. Ibid., p. 172.

26. Dennis Altman, *The Homosexualization of America* (Boston: Beacon Press, 1982), p. 175.

27. Dennis Altman, *AIDS in the Mind of America* (New York: Anchor Press/Doubleday, 1986), p. 159.

28. Johnston, op. cit., p. 168.

29. David P. McWhirter & Andrew M. Mattison, *The Male Couple: How Relationships Develop* (New York: Prentice-Hall, 1984).
30. Ibid., p. 291.
31. Baehr v. Miike, Slip Op. No. Civ. 91-1394 (Haw. Cir. Ct., December 3, 1996), aff'd, 950 P.2d 1234 (Haw. 1997).
32. Michael L. Closen & Carol R. Heise, "HIV–AIDS and the Non-Traditional Family: The Argument for State and Federal Judicial Recognition of Danish Same-Sex Marriages," *Nova Law Review, 16,* 809–845, 1992.
33. Tomas J. Philipson & Richard A. Posner, *Private Choices and Public Health: The AIDS Epidemic in an Economic Perspective* (Boston: Harvard University Press, 1993), p.117.
34. Philipson & Posner, op. cit., p. 148.
35. Ibid., p. 179.
36. Ibid.
37. Rofes, op. cit., p. 83.
38. Johnston, op. cit., p. 287.

Chapter 6

1. Dean Ornish, *Love and Survival: The Scientific Basis for the Healing Power of Intimacy* (New York: HarperCollins, 1998).
2. G. D. Travers Scott, in "Flexible Fidelity," Michael Lowenthal (Ed.), *Gay Men at the Millennium* (New York: Tarcher/Putnam, 1997), pp. 68–70.
3. G. J. Wagner, R. H. Remien, & A. Carballo-Dieguez, " 'Extramarital' Sex: Is There an Increased Risk for HIV Transmission?: A Study of Male Couples of Mixed HIV Status," *AIDS Education & Prevention 10,* 245–256, 1998.
4. Dan Woog, "Monogamy: Is it for Us." *Advocate,* p. 29, June 23, 1998.
5. Gloria Grening Wolk, *Cash for the Final Days: A Financial Guide for the Terminally Ill and Their Advisors* (Laguna Hills, CA: Bialkin Books, 1996).
6. Jean Baker Miller, *Toward a New Psychology of Women* (Boston: Beacon Press, 1976).
7. American Psychiatric Association, *Diagnostic and Statistical Manual of Mental Disorders,* 4th ed. (Washington, DC: Author, 1994), p. 665.
8. Cappy Capossella and Sheila Warnock, *Share the Care: How to Organize a Group to Care for Someone Who Is Seriously Ill* (New York: Simon & Schuster, 1995).
9. Peter D. Kramer, *Should You Leave?* (New York: Scribner, 1997).
10. Ibid.
11. Mira Kirshenbaum, *Too Good to Leave, Too Bad to Stay: A Step-by-Step Guide to Helping You Decide Whether to Stay In or Get Out of Your Relationship* (New York: Penguin Books, 1997), pp. 27–28.
12. Ibid, pp. 6–7.

Chapter 7

1. J. E. Bower, S. E. Taylor, et. al., "Cognitive Processing, Discovery of Meaning, CD4 Decline and AIDS Related Mortality Among Bereaved HIV-Seropositive Men," *Journal of Consulting and Clinical Psychology 66,* 979–986, December 1998.
2. Crixivan, by the way, was not necessarily more powerful than the earlier protease inhibitors, but it had advantages that made it more appealing to many patients.
3. Brian O'Connell, "I Never Thought I'd Live to 40," *Washington Blade,* p. 1, October 11, 1996.
4. Sheryl Gay Stolberg, "Despite New AIDS Drugs, Many Still Lose the Battle," *New York Times,* August 22, 1997.
5. Andrew Sullivan, "When Plagues End," *New York Times Magazine,* November 10, 1996.
6. Rando, Theresa A., (Ed.), *Loss and Anticipatory Grief* (Lexington, MA: Lexington Books).
7. Rofes, op. cit., p. 29.
8. David France, "Reprieve from AIDS Death Leaves Emotional Stresses," *New York Times,* October 11, 1998.
9. Stolberg, op. cit.
10. Kenneth J. Doka, *Disenfranchised Grief: Recognizing Hidden Sorrow* (San Francisco: Lexington Books, 1989).
11 Corless, I. B. "Modulated Mourning: The Grief and Mourning of Those Infected and Affected by HIV/AIDS," in Kenneth J. Doka (Ed.), *Living with Grief When Illness Is Prolonged* (Washington, DC: Hospice Foundation of America, 1997), p. 112.

Appendix A

1. Liz Seaton is Senior Counsel at the Human Rights Campaign; she previously worked as Associate Director of Legal Services at the Whitman-Walker Clinic, an HIV service provider in Washington, DC.

INDEX

Abandonment fears, 159
Acceptance of illness, 102–103
Activism, 188
Ad campaigns, 55
Addiction
  help for, 217
  to relationship, signs of, 161–162
  sexual, 42–44
  See also Substance abuse
Adversity, history of facing, 104–105
Affiliation, 151–152
Age and orgasm, 87
AID Atlanta, 177
AIDS and Its Metaphors (Sontag), 36
AIDS Counseling and Information
  Hotline, 95
AIDS Memorial Quilt, 171, 192, 193
Al-Anon, 217
Alaska, 144
Alcohol, 39–42, 76
Altman, Dennis, 130
"Altruism," 22–23
Ambivalence about relationship, 160
Androgenic steroidal agents, 63
Anger after recovery of lover, 168–
  170
Anonymous sex, 15–17, 42–43
Anticipatory grief, 174

Anxiety
  about relationship and fear of
    disclosure, 28–29
  in positive-negative relationship,
    61–64
  while awaiting test results, 127
Arsenequilt, Johanne, 135–136
Asking about HIV status, 134
Autonomy, fear of loss of, 152–153

B

Bareback sex, 106, 107–112, 129–
  130
Beardsell, Susan, 16
Beauty, emphasis on masculine, 53
Beneficiary, 212
Bonding and sense of community,
  151–152
Bruni, I. M., 70–71
"Bug chasers," 112
Burial directive, 213
Burnout, 101

C

Canada, 205
Capello, Dominic, 20

Capossella, Cappy, 153
Caretaker
    anger after recovery of lover, 168–
        170
    caring for, 101, 105
    stress and health of, 100
    taking on role of purposely, 79,
        80
Care team, 153–154
Cash for the Final Days (Wolk), 145
Casual sex, 15–17
Celibacy, 14–15
Chauncey, George, 11
Checklist for problematic
    relationships, 39
Checkups, regular, xiv, 65
Children
    arranging for care of, 212–213
    unborn, passing virus to, 196
Closen, Michael, 132
"Cocktail" drug, 88
Codependency, 80, 149
Coming out
    as HIV positive, 23
    HIV status and, 126
"Communal coping," 93, 104
"Community of choice," 189
Condoms
    negotiated safety and, 131
    putting on, 65
    refusal to use, 119
    as viral stopwatches, 87
    See also Bareback sex
Confidence, new sexual, 72–73
Confidentiality
    lawyer and, 204
    Monthly Social and, 11
Conservatorships, 211
Corea, Gina, 46
Corless, Inge, 189
Cost of AIDS, 145
Counseling and testing services,
    finding, xiv

Coupling as health benefit, 83–86,
    106
Crisis
    "fight-or-flight" response to, 78–
        79
    as opportunity for change, 35–36
    reacting to, 33
A Crisis of Meaning (Schwartzberg),
    90

D

Dating
    assertive approach to, 51–52
    meeting someone special, 49–50
    passive approach to, 48–49
    "Score on Four" model, 20–22
Dead, contacting, 186
Decision point in relationship, 135–
    136, 160–161
Denial, 157
Dependency vs. overdependency,
    152–153
Depression
    energy loss and, 56
    Lazarus syndrome and, 177
    as opportunistic disease, 84
    suicidal thoughts, 177–178
    time distortion and, 76
    violence and, 77
Diagnosis
    change and, 59–60
    hearing, 5
    initial rush to health after, 140
    as life-changing event, 36–38
    reacting to, 33
    as rite of passage, 89
    See also Growth, opportunity for
        after diagnosis
Differences between partners and
    discovery of serodiscordance,
    73–75
Differently abled, rights of, 2

*Directory of Legal Resources for People
    with AIDS and HIV,* 204
Disability insurance, 146–147
Discernment, 186
Disclosure
    effect on relationship, 22
    fear of, 13
    leap into trust and, 20
    legal issues and, 119
    listening to, 29–32
    moral judgments and, 36
    overview of, 9–10
    as "pattern of sexual caretaking,"
        22–23
    reaction to, 120–123
    relationship anxiety and, 28–29
    revealing or sharing compared to,
        23–25
    safer sex and, 66, 68
    withholding, 13–14
"Disclosure disincentive," 16–17
Discordant couple, 73–75
Disenfranchised grief, 188–190
Domestic partnership, 206
*Dry Bones Breathe: Gay Men Creating
    Post AIDS Identities and Cultures*
    (Rofes), 133, 174
Dumping emotions in relationship,
    94–95
Durable power of attorney, 210

E

Early detection, 157
Ebenhoch, Marc, 109
Elders, Jocelyn, 4
Emergency fund, 146
Emotions. *See* Anxiety; Depression;
    Grief; Guilt
Empathy and similarity, 82–83, 98,
    99, 116
Escándalo, 12–14
Exercise, 53

F

Family Medical Leave Act, 144
Family of partner, 189–190
Fear
    of abandonment, 159
    of disclosure, 13, 28–29
    of infecting negatives, 96–97
    of loss of autonomy, 152–153
    of rejection, 13, 15, 85, 97–99,
        119
Financial issues, 210–211
First date, 20
"Flexible Fidelity" (Scott), 142
Flirting vs. cruising, 49–50
Forrest Gump, 3–4
Fourth date, 21

G

The Gay and Lesbian National
    Hotline, 215
Gay bars, 40–41
Gay civil rights, start of, 2
*Gay New York: Gender, Urban Culture,
    and the Making of the Gay Male
    World 1890–1940* (Chauncey), 11
George Washington University
    Hospital, 11
"Glory holes," 42
Grief
    anticipatory, 174
    disenfranchised, 188–190
    men and, 190, 192
    serial, 127–129
    stages of, 191–192
    suffering and, 161
Growth, opportunity for after
    diagnosis
    change and, 36–38
    drinking, dating, and disclosing,
        34–35
    overview of, 33–34

Guilt
    dealing with, 184–188
    positive-positive relationship and,
        96–97
    of survivors, 124–127, 134

H

Hawaii, 131, 143–144
Health
    awareness of, 56–57
    disparity in status of between
        partners, 103
    healing power of love, 136–137
    initial rush to, 140
    responding to questions about,
        116
Health care power of attorney, 209
Health insurance, public vs. private,
    208–209
Hearing news of HIV-positive status,
    29–32
Heise, Carol, 132
Help, accepting, 103–104, 152–154
Hepatitis A and hepatitis B, 66
Heroic expectations, 25–28
HIV, redefinition of, 8
*HIV-Negative: How the Uninfected
    Are Affected by AIDS*
    (Johnston), 124–126, 127, 129,
    130, 134
HIV status
    asking about, 134
    financial benefit of knowing, 145–
        146
Ho, David, 110, 171–172
Homophobia, internalized, 35, 125–
    126
Honesty, 23
The Hopkins HIV Report (Pomerantz),
    72
Hotlines, 68, 95, 215–217

I

Ideal partner, list of qualities in, 18,
    25, 52–54
Identity
    common experience and shared,
        86
    construction of around disease, 5
    as survivor, 164–165
Impotency, 56
Infidelity, 95–96
Injection drug use, 41–42
Insurance
    disability, 146–147
    health, public vs. private, 208–209
    life, 145
Internet, 50–51
Interviews and interviewees, 6–7
Inter vivos trusts, 211
In the Shadow of the Epidemic (Odets),
    124, 126
Intimacy
    expressing, 106
    rushing, 94–95
    safer sex and, 123–124
    sexual abuse and, 44–48
    using easy sex as substitute for, 44
*The Invisible Epidemic: The Story of
    Women and AIDS* (Corea), 46
"Isaac Newton Theory of Love," 49
Isolation, 84–86

J

Job, starting new, 175–176, 178
Johnston, William, 124–126, 127,
    129, 130, 134

K

Kennedy, Joe, 182
Keogh, Peter, 16

King, Mark, 177
Kirshenbaum, Mira, 159, 160
Kramer, Peter, 154

L

"Last love"
    finding, 199
    looking for, 26–27
Lawyer
    communicating with, 204–205
    finding, 203–204
Lazarus syndrome
    anger of caregiver and, 169–170
    description of, 165
    Roemer and, 172
    uncertainty and, 177–178
Leaving relationship
    legal issues, 206–207
    "till death do us part" and, 160–161
Legal issues
    disclosure, 119
    financial transactions, 210–211
    marriage, 205–207
    powers of attorney, 147
    property rights, 211–212
    transmission of HIV, 207–208
    See also Lawyer
Lew, Mike, 46, 48
Life insurance, 145
Lifespan and spread of disease, 87
Listening to Prozac (Kramer), 154
Living will, 208
Location of search for Mr. Right, 52
Long-term relationship
    end of, 155–160
    positive-positive, 138–143, 147–150
    sex in, 61–62
Loss of partner, surviving, 164–165

Love
    after loss, 190, 192–194
    healing power of, 136–137
    See also Intimacy
Love American Style, 2
Love and Survival: The Scientific Basis
        for the Healing Power of Intimacy
        (Ornish), 137

M

Magnetic couple, 79–81
The Male Couple (McWhirter and
        Mattison), 131
Mann, David, 37
Marriage and legal protections,
        205–207. See also Same-sex
        marriage
Medical issues
    checkups, regular, xiv, 65
    disability insurance, 3
    early detection, 157
    Family Medical Leave Act, 144
    health care power of attorney, 209
    health insurance, 208–209
    impotency, 56
    See also Caretaker; Depression;
        Diagnosis; Health; Protease
        inhibitors
Meeting someone special, 49–50
Menstruation as illness, 85
Methadone, 41–42
Miller, Jean Baker, 151
Moneyham, Linda, 178
Money issues, 144–147
Monogamy
    expanded, 141
    in negative-negative relationship,
        129–131
    variations of, 142
    See also Same-sex marriage
Monthly Social, 10–12, 17–18

N

Narcotics Anonymous group for
    HIV-positive men, 37–38
National AIDS Hotline, 68
National Clinical Trials Hotline, 217
National PEP Hotline, 68
National Prevention Information
    Network, 216
National Sexually Transmitted
    Diseases (STD) Hotline, 216
Negative-negative relationship
    bareback sex in, 129–130
    expectations of, 129
    monogamy in, 129–131
    negotiated safety in, 131
    overview of, 118–119
    personal ads and, 122–123
    reasons for, 127
    safer sex and, 123–124, 129
Negotiated safety, 131
Network of support, creating, 80–81
Nimmons, David, 22
Nurturance
    men and, 150–152
    as mutual, 154

O

Odets, Walt, 124, 126
O'Hara, Scott, 55
Online chat rooms, 50–51
Open relationship, 141, 142
Optimism and will to live, 179–183
Oral sex, 65–66
Orgasm and age, 87
Ornish, Dean, 137

P

Parks, Lamar, 37
"Partnership agreements," 206–207
"Pass," ability to, 113

Peers, finding, 28
PEP (postexposure prophylaxis), 68–
    71
Personal ads
    of negative persons, 122–123,
        128–129
    of positive persons, 18–19
PETS DC, 146
Philipson, Tomas, 132–133
Policing Public Sex (O'Hara), 55
Pomerantz, Richard J., 72
Positive-negative relationship
    anxiety, HIV, and sex in, 61–63
    discordant couple, 73–75
    risk and responsibility in, 63–64
    role confusion and power
        struggles in, 77–81
    safer sex and, 64–73
    time warp, taking control of in,
        75–77
Positive parties, 10–12, 17–18
Positive-positive relationship
    bareback sex in, 107–112
    biology as biography, 88–89
    common experience and shared
        identity in, 86
    coupling as health benefit, 83–86
    discordance in, 100–106
    fear of infecting negatives and,
        96–97
    fear of rejection and, 97–99
    intensity and speed of, 89–90
    long-term, 138–143, 147–150
    negative reasons for, 90–94
    perceptions of risk, differing,
        106–107
    relief from dating tension in, 86–
        88
    similarity and empathy in, 82–83,
        98, 99, 116
Posner, Richard, 132–133
Postexposure prophylaxis (PEP), 68–
    71

Powell, Colin, 113
Power struggles, 77–81
POZ magazine's Life Expo health
     fair, 59
Preemptive therapy, 70–71
Prejudice about positives, 96
Pride Institute, 42, 217
Privacy, invasion of, 16
Probate procedures, 211–212
Property rights, 211–212
Prostitution, 46
Protcase inhibitors
     "cocktail" drug, 88
     as morning-after treatment,
          69–70
     perceived effectiveness of, 108,
          109
     promises and warnings of, 174
     research on, 171–172
     side effects of, 176–177
"Protease moment," 174–176
"Psychosocial" problems and risk,
     47
Psychotherapy: An Erotic Relationship
     (Mann), 37
Public educational campaigns, 4
Public sex, 15, 17

Q

Queer as Folk, 64, 120–121

R

"Raw sex," 106, 107–112
Reduction in sexual activity, 61–63
Reinfection, 107
Reinventing self, 180–182
Rejection, fear of
     celibacy and, 15
     isolation and, 85
     positive-positive relationship and,
          97–99

refusal to use condoms and, 119
     withholding disclosure and, 13
Relationship
     healthy, mature, signs of, 114
     impediments to, 48
     problematic, 38–39
Relationship addiction, signs of,
     161–162
Reno, Janet, 179
Resilience, 48
Retirement planning, 146
Revealing compared to disclosing,
     23–25
Risk
     bareback sex, 107–112
     perception of, 72–73
     protease inhibitors and, 108, 109
     of sexual behaviors, 67
     viral elite, 106–107, 112–113
Roemer, Jerry, 82, 171–173, 178,
     201
Rofes, Eric, 133, 174
Role confusion, 77–81
Role modeling, 28

S

Safer sex
     discarding practices of, 123–124
     going beyond, 4–5
     guidelines for, 65–68
     positive-negative relationship, 64–73
     substance abuse and, 40
Safer-sex parties, 17
Same-sex marriage
     barriers to, 143
     in Hawaii, 131, 143–144
     public health and economic
          arguments for, 132–134
     states banning, 205–206
Schnell, Daniel, 22
Schwartzberg, Steven, 90
"Score on Four" model, 20–22

Scott, G. D. Travers, 142
Screening, annual, recommendations
    for, xiv
Second date, 21
Self, reinventing, 180–182
Self-destructive behavior, 178
Serodiscordance
    differences between partners and
        discovery of, 73–75
    role confusion and power
        struggles, 77–81
    safer sex and, 64–73
    time, understanding, 75–77
Seroharmonious, 82
Sex. *See also* Safer sex
    anonymous, 15–16, 42–43
    bareback, 106, 107–112, 129–130
    in long-term relationship, 61–62
    with love vs. without love, 3
    oral, 65–66
    public, 15, 17
    as substitute for intimacy, 44
    unprotected or unsafe, 6–7, 109
Sexual abuse, 44–48
Sexual compulsivity or addiction,
    42–44
Share the Care (Capossella and
    Warnock), 153
Sharing, 24
Should You Leave? (Kramer), 154
Social events, 11. *See also* Monthly
    Social
Social Security, 210
Sodomy laws, 207
Sontag, Susan, 36
*The Soul Beneath the Skin: The Unseen
    Hearts and Habits of Gay Men*
    (Nimmons), 22
South Carolina, 144
Sperm donation, 196
Springing guardianship, 213
State law, 203
Staying well, 176–179

Stein, Michael, 84
Stigma
    acceptance of, 25
    identity and, 5
    knowledge of positive status and,
        35–36
    moving beyond, 55–58
Stonewall riots, 2
Stress, reducing, 116
"Stress inoculation," 101
Suarez, Troy P., 72
Substance abuse, 39–42, 76
Suffering, 155
Suicidal thoughts, 177–178
Sullivan, Andrew, 173
Support groups, 42–43, 44, 94–95
Support system
    creating, 80–81
    sharing, 105–106
Survivor
    of childhood abuse, 46
    guilt of, 124–127, 134
    of HIV, identity as, 164–165

T

Tainted love, xiii, xv, 55–58
"Talk, Test, Test, Talk" model, 131
Testamentary guardianship, 213
Testosterone, 56, 61, 63
Third date, 21
Time warp, taking control of, 75–77
Too Good to Leave, Too Bad to Stay
    (Kirshenbaum), 159, 160
Toward a New Psychology of Women
    (Miller), 151
Transmission of HIV, criminalization
    of, 207–208
Treatment hotlines, 216–217
Trust
    hearing disclosure and, 31–32
    intimacy and, 44–48
    leap into with disclosure, 20

U

Undetectable viral load, perceptions
    of, 72–73
Unprotected sex, 109
Unsafe sex practices, 6–7

V

Vaccinations, 66
Vaccine trials, 138
Vermont, 205
Viatical company ads, 145
Victims No Longer (Lew), 46
Vietnam, war in, 2–4
Violence, 77
Viral elite, 106–107, 112–113
Viral load, 72–73

W

Warnock, Sheila, 153
Washington Blade, 71, 188
Washington Post, 189

Websites
    AIDS Memorial Quilt, 193
    author, 50
    chat rooms and bulletin boards,
        50
    contacting dead, 186
    counseling and testing services,
        xiv
    gay community centers, 95
    national AIDS organizations, 218
    parties/socials, 18
    personal ads, 19, 50
    positive-negative relationships, 62
    vaccine trials, 138
"When Plagues End" (Sullivan), 173
White, Ryan, 37
Wolk, Gloria Grening, 145
Women and HIV, 194–199
Worried well, 123–129

Y

Yellow Light Rule, 31–32

ABOUT THE AUTHORS

Michael Mancilla, MSW, LICSW, is a Washington, DC-based psychotherapist who specializes in working with individuals, couples, and families affected by HIV/AIDS. He is a frequent presenter at national and international conferences. Mr. Mancilla's story of the impact of HIV on his relationship was the subject of a *Washington Post Magazine* article and a CNN documentary, and was cited in a front-page story in *The New York Times.* He can be contacted via his website at *www.hivandrelationships.com.*

Lisa Troshinsky is a writer and editor in Washington, DC. She has reported on HIV/AIDS and gay and lesbian issues for the *Washington Blade,* the *Houston Chronicle,* and United Press International.

2 6/95